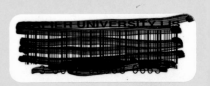

Depression in Old Age

Detta är en gåva från

NOVO NORDISK PHARMA AB

Depression in Old Age

CORNELIUS L.E. KATONA

Professor of Psychiatry of the Elderly
University College London Medical School, UK

JOHN WILEY & SONS

Chichester · New York · Brisbane · Toronto · Singapore

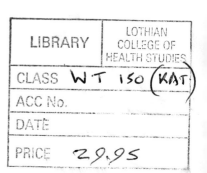

Other Wiley Editorial Offices

John Wiley & Sons, Inc., 605 Third Avenue,
New York, NY 10158-0012, USA

Jacaranda Wiley Ltd, 33 Park Road, Milton,
Queensland 4064, Australia

John Wiley & Sons (Canada) Ltd, 22 Worcester Road,
Rexdale, Ontario M9W 1L1, Canada

John Wiley & Sons (SEA) Pte Ltd, 37 Jalan Pemimpin #05-04,
Block B, Union Industrial Building, Singapore 2057

Library of Congress Cataloging-in-Publication Data

Karona, C. L. E. (Cornelius L. E.), 1954–
    Depression in old age / Cornelius L. E. Katona.
        p.   cm.
    Includes bibliographical references and index.
    ISBN 0 471 94308 8
    1. Depression in old age.   I. Title.
RC537.5.K38   1994
618.97'68527—dc20   93-46294
                                           CIP

British Library Cataloguing in Publication Data

A catalogue record for this book is available from the British Library

ISBN 0 471 94308 8

Typeset in 10/12pt Times by Mathematical Composition Setters Ltd, Salisbury, Wiltshire
Printed and bound in Great Britain by Biddles Ltd, Guildford and King's Lynn

To the memory of my father
Paul Katona

Contents

Acknowledgements

Earlier versions of some of the material in this volume have appeared in *Current Opinion in Psychiatry* **3**, 512–515 (1990); *The Nordic Journal of Psychiatry* **47**(28), 53–8 (1993); *Dysthymic Disorder* (edited by S.W. Burton and H.S. Akiskal; London, Gaskell Press, 1990); *International Review of Psychiatry* (in press); *Clinics in Geriatric Medicine* **8**, 275–287 (1992); *Treatment and Care in Old Age Psychiatry* (edited by R. Levy, R. Howard and A. Burns; Petersfield, Wrightson Biomedical Publishing); and *Recent Advances in Old Age Psychiatry* 2 (edited by T.H.D. Arie; Edinburgh, Churchill Livingstone); all appear here in revised and updated versions by kind permission of the copyright holders.

Of the rating scales reproduced in the Appendix to Chapter 2, the Geriatric Depression Scale first appeared in the *Journal of Psychiatric Research*, and the SELFCARE-D in the *International Journal of Geriatric Psychiatry*. The BASDEC is published by Merck Pharmaceuticals.

Figure 6.1 is taken from a paper by James Lindesay in the *International Journal of Geriatric Psychiatry* and Table 7.3 is adapted from a paper by Robin and Lorna Morris in the same journal, to all of whom I extend my thanks.

I owe a great debt of thanks to Drs Gary Bell, Emily Finch and Ros Ramsay, who co-authored earlier published versions of some of the material in the book. Dr Bob Baldwin made many constructive criticisms on a draft typescript of the whole book; the final version would have been much the worse without his help. I would also like to thank Debbie Harrington who typed much of the text with more patience than I deserved.

My greatest debt of gratitude is to the many patients who have taught me that one should never regard depression as either inevitable or untreatable, and that when it remits sufferers can change more than I would have thought possible.

Introduction

Depression in old age is common and disabling. It is associated with increased mortality, both by suicide and by natural causes. As the proportion of the population that is old or very old increases throughout the developed world, so too will the size of the clinical problem of depression in old age.

The appropriate management of such depression is bedevilled by many difficulties. It is under-detected and even where identified it is all too seldom appropriately treated. Reluctance to treat older people with depression stems from the fundamental misconceptions that it is an inevitable consequence of aging and that the hazards of its treatment outweigh those of the condition itself. The intention of this book is to contribute to the elimination of these misconceptions.

Academic research in the field of depression in old age has come of age. The burgeoning of such research, particularly in Britain, the United States and Australia, has generated a wealth of information concerning its epidemiology, appropriate management and prognosis. As a result, depression in old age has attained a level of importance equal to that of the dementia, which until quite recently were seen as the main, if not the only, legitimate areas for research and service development in old age psychiatry.

This book is a distillate of the research information currently available on depression in old age which attempts to identify some of the questions as yet unanswered as well as summarising the answers we already have. It should be a useful source for those currently engaged in research in the area and those thinking of undertaking such research. It should also provide guidance on the detection and management of depression for clinicians (with backgrounds in medicine, nursing, psychology and allied professions) working with elderly people.

1 Clinical Features of Depression in Old Age

THE PRESENTING SYMPTOMS OF DEPRESSION IN OLD AGE

The presentation of depression in old age is often less obvious and straightforward than in younger subjects. The pathoplastic effects of aging and the different characteristics of birth cohorts as they age are both major influences on the clinical features of depression. Presentations which minimise depression but focus on somatic complaints and hypochondriasis are far more frequently found than in younger age groups. Cognitive deficits (which may or may not resolve with recovery from the depression) are also common features of depression in later life.

Shulman (1989) emphasises the fact that sadness is far from the commonest presentation of depression in the elderly—'neurotic' presentations with generalised anxiety and subjective complaints of nervousness and irritability being far more frequent. The distraught, 'importuning' elderly depressed patient may present a particularly difficult challenge to the tolerance as well as the diagnostic skills of the clinician.

Brodaty et al. (1991) point out that, though several clinical features (such as anxiety, preoccupation with physical symptoms, retardation, fatiguability, self-reproach, suicidality and insomnia) have been claimed to be more common in elderly than in younger depressed patients, the systematic comparison by Gurland (1976) found only an excess of hypochondriacal symptoms, and that by Musetti et al.(1989) virtually no differences at all apart from a slight excess in retardation.

More typical of the literature is the classic paper by Brown et al.(1984) on involutional melancholia. They examined 31 patients with depression of first onset after the age of 50 (the 'involutional' group) and compared them both with younger depressed patients and with patients of similar age but with a past history of depression earlier in life. Regardless of age at first onset, older patients had greater initial insomnia, agitation and hypochondriasis but less depersonalisation, suicidal intent and loss of libido. The involutional group had less guilt but more somatic anxiety, anorexia and hypochondriasis than subjects of similar age with earlier first onset. Positive family psychiatric history was also less common in the involutional group.

A more recent primary care based study by Oxman et al. (1990) examined symptom pattern in older (60 +) and younger (18–59) patients fulfilling Research

Diagnostic Criteria (RDC: Spitzer and Endicott 1978) for minor depressive disorder. In this relatively mildly ill sample, the only significant age-related differences found were in the following three symptoms, all of which were less common in the older group: irritability (63% vs 95%); feeling pushed to get things done (47% vs 91%); and loss of interest (37% vs 73%). In a similar comparison between older and younger outpatient referrals to a psychiatric service fulfilling DSM III (American Psychiatric Association 1980) criteria for unipolar major depressive episode, Brodaty et al. (1991) found that subjects aged 60 and over showed a higher rate of delusions, agitation, altered appetite, hypersomnia and guilt.

These studies suggest that the degree of difference found between older and younger subjects may depend crucially on the inclusion criteria used. Criteria for diagnosing depression designed for use in a younger adult population may be inappropriate for elderly subjects. In a community sample of 1529 subjects aged 60 and over in Finland, Kivela et al. (1989) were able to identify only 42 (2.7%) fulfilling DSM III criteria for major depression. However, a further 21 (1.4%) fulfilled criteria for atypical depression, and as many as 199 (13.0%) for dysthymic disorder, otherwise known as chronic mild depression. The overall symptomatology was of similar severity in the major depression and dysthymia groups, who also did not differ in mean age. Sadness, paranoid symptoms, loss of interest, loss of weight and depersonalisation were, however, commoner in subjects with major depression. This suggests that the severe/mild distinction, though important in deciding on appropriate management in individual cases, is not as applicable in older subjects as it is in their younger counterparts. In view of the overlap between depressive symptomatology and the changes in sleep, appetite and somatic symptoms associated with normal aging, it may be more useful to approach the delineation of clinical features of depression in old age by studying a broad range of elderly patients with and without clinically relevant depression than by making formal comparisons with younger subjects.

Kivela and Pahkala (1988a,b,c) have done precisely that in a series of studies based on the community sample referred to above. They identified a number of individual symptoms from the Hamilton Depression Rating Scale (HDRS; Hamilton 1967) that were particularly frequent in their depressed subjects, and also identified some sex differences. Initial and middle insomnia, loss of interest and low mood were commoner in depressed men; and anxiety, somatic symptoms, initial insomnia, loss of interest and depressed mood in depressed women. Though loss of libido was common in depressed subjects of both sexes, it was also frequently found in the absence of depression. In a factor analysis of the HDRS items, a factor structure somewhat different from that reported in younger patients (e.g. Hamilton 1967; Paykel et al. 1971) emerged. The first factor (depressed mood with loss of interest, accounting for 18.7% of the total variance) was similar to that in previous studies, but the second (somatic anxiety with hypochondriasis, 7.9%) was more in keeping with the finding by Brown et al. (1984) of prominent hypochondriasis and somatic anxiety in involutional melancholia. The other factors identified by Kivela et al. were guilt with sleep disturbance and loss of insight (6.7%), and suicidal ideation with gastrointestinal symptoms (6.1%). The factor structure was, however, quite different when male and female subjects were analysed separately: in particular, the cluster of somatic and hypochondriacal symptoms was evident in women but not in men.

Kivela and Pahkala (1988a) also examined physician-detected symptoms and signs in this population, and revealed a further accentuation of the sex differences described above. While both depressed men and depressed women exhibited sleep disturbance, fatigue and loss of interest; worrying, crying, helplessness, hopelessness and suicidal ideation were much more frequently detected in depressed women.

Good et al. (1987) used a varimax factor analysis of HDRS items to demonstrate four factor groupings which have clinical relevance in the depressed elderly—depression, anxiety, cognitive impairment and psychosomatic disorder. High scores on the depression factor were observed to be frequently associated with high scores on the psychosomatic disorder factor, confirming the importance of somatic symptoms in depression in the elderly. Gurland (1976) also reported an increase in somatic concern in the depressed elderly.

A small study by Kramer-Ginsberg et al. (1989) focused on the importance of hypochondriacal symptomatology in a more severely ill sample (depressed inpatients) than that studied by Kivela and Pahkala. In their sample of 70 consecutive depressed admissions, 60% scored positively on the hypochondriasis item of the HDRS. Hypochondriasis was not, in this sample, associated with severity of depression or with suicidality.

Downes et al. (1988) used Guttman scalar analyses to confirm the hierarchical organisation of depressive symptoms in old age. Not only were a number of symptoms particularly common, but rarer symptoms were virtually never present in the absence of the commoner ones. Downes et al. divided their symptoms into affective and somatic; affective symptoms at the top of the hierarchy were worrying, crying, life not being worth living and finding the future frightening; top-rated somatic symptoms were subjective slowing, listlessness and a cluster related to hypochondriasis.

Fredman et al. (1989) examined depressive symptoms in a large community sample of 1606 subjects aged 60 or over participating in the ECA-Piedmont Health Survey, using a checklist based on DSM III and achieving a response rate of 90%. Sleep disturbance was present in 14.8% and thoughts of death in 10%. Other common symptoms were fatigue, agitation or retardation, appetite disturbance and concentration difficulties. Depressed mood was present in only 5% and loss of libido in 1.4%. Given the importance of depressed mood in reaching a DSM III diagnosis of major depression, it is hardly surprising that its prevalence in this sample was only 2.7%.

DEPRESSION AND COGNITIVE DYSFUNCTION

Prominent cognitive dysfunction is the essential clinical feature in the minority of elderly depressed patients with 'depressive pseudodementia', though the term is by no means used consistently (Bulbena and Berrios 1986). Kral and Emery (1989) identified 44 such patients (mean age 76.5 years) with rapid onset of loss of interest, slowing, poor concentration, and poor memory and orientation coexistent with severe depression characterised by self-depreciation, guilt, suicidal ideas and loss of appetite. Though all subjects responded well to antidepressant treatment, showing remission of cognitive deficits as well as depressive symptoms, follow-up for an average of eight years revealed that 89% subsequently developed dementia of the Alzheimer type.

Though the subgroup of elderly depressed patients with such gross but reversible cognitive impairments is well established, the question of abnormalities in intellectual function in elderly depressed patients without frank pseudo-dementia has received relatively little attention. La Rue (1989), using the Fuld Object Memory Evaluation (Fuld 1981), found poorer overall performance in depressed than in control elderly subjects, but failed to confirm earlier findings (Hart et al. 987) of specific deficits of retrieval from memory in old age depression. Miller et al. (1991) noted that prior studies have been flawed by the inclusion of patients on antidepressants and other treatments, small sample sizes and unvalidated neuropsychological tests. In a non-elderly sample, they found no depression-related abnormalities in the Luria–Nebraska neuropsychological battery (Golden et al. 1980) and no relationship within the depressed sample between test performance and severity of depression.

However, Cipolli et al. (1990), who examined memory function in a group of elderly depressed and non-depressed subjects with grossly intact cognitive function, found severity of depression to correlate with degree of deficit on tests of both acquisition/recall and delayed memory. Emery and Breslau (1989) found significant differences in language processing between depressed and healthy elderly subjects, depression being associated with reduced linguistic complexity. In a large sample of middle-aged patients (mean age 55.5), Sackeim et al. (1992) found pronounced deficits in performance IQ in depressed subjects, though depression was not associated with any reduction in verbal IQ. When patients were tested again two months after treatment with ECT, some overall improvement in IQ score was noted but the verbal-performance deficit was unaltered. The authors considered that the IQ deficits they reported could not be explained in terms of depressive retardation, since removal of time constraints did not affect the results. In a specifically elderly sample, Abas et al. (1990) found that depression was associated with reductions in pattern and spatial recognition tasks and improved only partially with clinical recovery. The authors concluded that depression was associated with partially irreversible 'faulty effortful processing'.

There thus appears to be quite an impressive body of evidence to suggest that deficits in language and memory functioning, as well as more complex cognitive processing, do occur within depression in old age. Such deficits may not be explicable either in terms of depressive retardation or lack of motivation, and may also not be fully reversible. The distinction between depressive pseudodementia and uncomplicated depression in old age may thus not be as clear-cut as previously thought.

SUBTYPES OF DEPRESSION IN OLD AGE

Conventional subtypings of depression may, as has already been mentioned in passing, be much less appropriate in older subjects. Perhaps the best-documented subdivision of depression in younger patients is the endogenous/non-endogenous dichotomy. This concept has been operationalised by Carney et al. (1965) as the Newcastle Depression Index (NDI). Most diagnostic systems, including the RDC, DSM III and DSM IIIR (American Psychiatric Association 1987), incorporate similar concepts of endogenicity. Burvill et al. (1989) found that 82% of 103 elderly depressed patients treated by psychiatrists were 'endogenous' on the NDI, a much larger proportion than would be expected in a younger adult population. They also found that, using DSM III, approximately one-third each had delusional depression, melancholia and major depression without melancholia—a result very similar to that reported by Conwell et al. (1989). Furthermore, Gallagher-Thompson et al. (1992) have reported that, in elderly patients, level of agreement between alternative definitions of endogenicity was generally poor, with the exception of RDC and DSM IIIR, which were in close agreement. Little relationship was found between endogenicity and demographic and clinical variables including severity.

Alexopoulos (1989) suggests that depression in old age might usefully be classified in terms of age at first onset. He reviews evidence suggesting that subjects with a first onset of depression after the age of 60 (late onset, LO) are characterised by greater CT scan abnormalities, less frequently positive family history, poor treatment response and greater risk of both progression to dementia and earlier mortality than those with a past history of depression earlier in life (EO). Evidence for the biological and prognostic distinctness of LO are reviewed in subsequent chapters. It ishowever worth noting at this point that a number of recent studies have compared symptom pattern and family history in elderly depressed subjects with LO and EO. Conwell et al. (1989) found that LO and EO subjects did not differ in rate of melancholia or psychosis, or in overall severity, but that those with LO were less likely to have a positive family history, and had longer hospital stays with more residual symptoms. Burvill et al. (1989), however, found their LO subjects to have more severe illnesses but not to differ in family history or likelihood of recent adverse life events. There was a trend for psychosis to be commoner in EO. LO subjects had greater cognitive impairment, as predicted by Alexopoulos (1989), though this might have been a reflection of their greater median age (75–79 vs 60–64). A higher likelihood of positive family history in elderly depressed patients with EO was also the only differ-ence (apart from a higher rate of personality abnormalities) between the two groups found by Brodaty et al. (1991). Herrmann et al. (1989) also found positive family history to be associated more frequently with EO (80%) than with LO (28%) but found no other differences related either to age at onset or chronological age. Kivela and Pahkala (1988c), however, while not making comparisons based on age at onset, found that their chronologically older (70 +) community-detected depressed subjects had more severe symptoms, particularly depressed mood and somatic symptoms, than those aged 60–69. No significant differences in symptom pattern, degree of cognitive impairment, treatment response or even family history were found by Greenwald and Kramer–Ginsberg (1988).

Baldwin (1992) has made a comprehensive review of the question of whether delusional depression in old age should be regarded as a clinically distinct subtype. He points out that the prevalence of delusions within samples of elderly depressed patients depends crucially on the method of sampling. Whereas Kivela and Pahkala (1988c) found that only 1% of a community-drawn sample had depressive delusions, samples of elderly depressed patients drawn from specialist psychiatric referrals have reported prevalence rates for delusions ranging between 24% (Murphy 1983) and 53% (Post 1972). Baldwin's own study reported a prevalence of 34% in a sample of 134 consecutive depressed referrals to a catchment old age psychiatry service. Within the sample, delusions were associated with greater severity of depression and with a relative excess of males. The predominant delusions were persecutory and hypochondriacal. No relationship was found in this study between the presence of delusions and age at first onset, though a similar and earlier study by Meyers and Greenberg (1986) found that in women (though not in men) LO subjects were more frequently deluded. Baldwin also found deluded subjects not to have a significantly different prognosis, though the presence of delusions tended to 'run true' in subsequent episodes, seldom occurring in subjects who had not previously been deluded. Baldwin (1992) concluded that supportive evidence for accepting delusional depression in old age as a distinct clinical entity was as yet limited.

DEPRESSION IN DEMENTIA

Wragg and Jeste (1989) reviewed several studies of the phenomenology and prevalence of depressive symptoms and depressive illness in patients with established Alzheimer's disease. The studies they examined used widely varying methodologies, though most relied on clinical ratings alone or scales designed for use in younger cognitively unimpaired adults. Depressed mood was recorded in 0–87% of subjects (median 41%) and depressive disorder (including dysthymia) in 0–86% (median 19%). In most studies, depressed mood was commoner in the Alzheimer's disease subjects than in healthy elderly controls. More recently, two studies (Greenwald et al. 1989; Rovner et al. 1989), using a combination of semi-structured interviews and rating scales, have reported prevalence rates for major depression of 17% and 11% respectively, in patients with Alzheimer's disease. Rovner et al. (1989) found depression to be associated with more severe impairment, both cognitively and in daily living skills. Greenwald et al. (1989) found more frequent self-pity and rejection sensitivity, but less worrying, anhedonia and sleep and appetite disturbances in patients with coexisting depression and dementia than in those with pure depressive illnesses. They further noted that antidepressant treatment was associated with some improvement in cognitive function as well as resolution of the depressive symptoms.

BEREAVEMENT

Symptom patterns in elderly bereaved subjects with and without clear-cut depressive illnesses have been examined by Zisook et al. (1987) in a cohort of 189 widows and widowers (mean age 60.4) two months after their bereavement. Disbelief and yearning were experienced by the majority of subjects, with numbness, self-reproach and anger being less frequently noted. The main clinical features of prolonged active grief were anxiety, somatisation, interpersonal sensitivity and depressed mood; 28% of the subjects fulfilled DSM III criteria for major depression. An interesting short paper by Herrmann and Grek (1988) serves as a reminder that demented patients can experience major emotional and behavioural responses to the bereavements they frequently experience. They report two cases of 'delusional double mourning' in moderately demented subjects who, following the death of a spouse, developed the fixed delusion that a parent had also very recently died.

CONCLUSIONS

It is clear that depression in old age presents with quite different symptom patterns that represent a considerable diagnostic challenge. In particular, somatic symptoms and cognitive deficits are frequently apparent and depressed mood may be conspicuous by its absence. The presentation of depression may be particularly confusing in the contexts of bereavement and of dementia. The subtyping of depression using concepts derived in a younger population is unsatisfactory. The most promising approach to a specific subclassification of depression in old age is that based on age at first onset. More research (examining biological correlates, treatment–response and outcome) is needed to validate or refute it.

REFERENCES

Abas MA, Sahakian BJ and Levy R (1990) Neuropsychological deficits and CT scan changes it elderly depressives. *Psychological Medicine* **20**, 507–20.
Alexopoulos GS (1989) Late-life depression and neurological brain disease. *International Journal of Geriatric Psychiatry* **4**, 181–90.

American Psychiatric Association (1980) *Diagnostic and Statistical Manual of Mental Disorders* (3rd edn). Washington, American Psychiatric Association.

American Psychiatric Association (1987) *Diagnostic and Statistical Manual of Mental Disorders* (3rd edn, revised). Washington, American Psychiatric Association.

Baldwin RC (1992) The nature, prevalence and frequency of depressive delusions. in Katona C and Levy R (eds) *Delusions and Hallucinations in Old Age*, Ch. 8, pp. 97–114. London, Gaskell.

Brodaty H, Peters K, Boyce P et al. (1991) Age and depression. *Journal of Affective Disorders* 23, 137–49.

Brown RP, Sweeney J, Loutsch E et al. (1984) Involutional melancholia revisited. *American Journal of Psychiatry* 137, 439–44.

Bulbena A and Berrios GE (1986) Pseudodementia: facts and figures. *British Journal of Psychiatry* 148, 81–4.

Burvill PW, Hall WD, Stampfer HG and Emmerson JP (1989) A comparison of early-onset and late-onset depressive illness in the elderly. *British Journal of Psychiatry* 155, 673–9.

Carney MWP, Roth M and Garside RF (1965) The diagnosis of depressive syndromes and the pediction of ECT response. *British Journal of Psychiatry* 111, 659–74.

Cipolli C, Neri M, Andermarcher E et al. (1990) Self-rating and objective memory testing of normal and depressed elderly. *Aging Milano* 2, 39–48.

Conwell C, Nelson JC, Kim KM and Mazure CM (1989) Depression in late life: age of onset as marker of a subtype. *Journal of Affective Disorders* 17, 189–95.

Downes JJ, Davis ADM and Copeland JRM (1988) Organisation of depressive symptoms in the elderly population: hierarchal patterns and Guttman scales. *Psychology and Aging* 3, 367–74.

Emery OB and Breslau LD (1989) Language deficits in depression: comparions with SDAT and normal aging. *Journal of Gerontology* 44, M85–92.

Fredman L, Schoenbach VJ, Kaplan BH et al. (1989) The association between depressive symptoms and mortality among older participants in the Epidemiologic Catchment Area—Piedmont Health Survey. *Journal of Gerontology* 44, S149–56.

Fuld PA (1981) *The Fuld Object—Memory Evaluation*. Chicago, Stoelting Instrument Company.

Gallagher-Thompson D, Futterman A, Hanley-Paterson P et al.(1992) Endogenous depression in the elderly: prevalence and agreement among measures. *Journal of Consulting and Clinical Psychology* 60, 300–3.

Golden CJ, Hammeke T and Purish A (1980) *A Manual for the Administration and Interpretation of the Luria–Nebraska Neuropsychological Battery*. Los Angeles, Western Psychological Services.

Good WR, Vlachonikolis I, Griffiths P and Griffiths RA (1987) The structure of depressive symptoms in the elderly. *British Journal of Psychiatry* 150, 463–70.

Greenwald BS and Kramer-Ginsberg E (1988) Age at onset in geriatric depression: relationship to clinical variables. *Journal of Affective Disorders* 15, 61–8.

Greenwald BS, Kramer-Ginsberg E, Marin DB et al. (1989) Dementia with coestent major depression. *American Journal of Psychiatry* 146, 1472–8.

Gurland BJ (1976) The comparative frequency of depression in various adult age groups. *Journal of Gerontology* 31, 283–92.

Hamilton M (1967) Development of a rating scale for primary depressive illness. *British Journal of Social and Clinical Psychology* 6, 278–96.

Hart RP, Kwentus JA, Hamer RM and Taylor JF (1987) Selective reminding procedure in depression and dementia. *Psychology and Aging* 2, 111–15.

Herrmann N and Grek A (1988) Delusional double mourning: a complication of bereavement in dementia. *Canadian Journal of Psychiatry* 33, 851–2.

Herrmann N, Lieff S and Silberfield M (1989) The effect of age of onset on depression in the elderly. *Journal of Geriatric Psychiatry and Neurology* 2, 182-7.

Kivela S-L and Pahkala K (1988a) Clinician-rated symptoms and signs of depression in aged Finns. *International Journal of Social Psychiatry* 34, 274-84.

Kivela S-L and Pahkala K (1988b) Factor structure of the Hamilton rating scale for depression among deressed elderly Finns. *Zeitschrift für Psychologie* 196, 389-99.

Kivela S-L and Pahkala K (1988c) Symptoms of depression old people in Finland. *Zeitschrift für Gerontologie* 21, 257-63.

Kivela S-L, Pahkala K and Eronen P (1989) Depressive symptoms and signs that differentiate major and atypical depression from dysthymic disorder in elderly Finns. *International Journal of Geriatric Psychiatry* 4, 79-85.

Kral VA and Emery OB (1989) Long-term follow-up of depressive pseudodementia of the aged. *Canadian Journal of Psychiatry* 34, 445-6.

Kramer-Ginsberg E, Greenwald BS, Aisen PS and Brod-Miller C (1989) Hypochondriasis in the elderly depressed. *Journal of the American Geriatric Society* 37, 507-10.

La Rue A (1989) Patterns of performance on the Fuld Object Memory Evaluation in elderly inpatients with depression or dementia. *Journal of Clinical and Experimental Neuropsychology* 11, 409-22.

Meyers BS and Greenberg R (1986) Late-life delusional depression. *Journal of Affective Disorders* 11, 133-7.

Miller LS, Faustman WO, Moses JA and Csernansky JG (1991) Evaluating cognitive impairment in depression with the Luria-Nebraska Neuropsychological Battery: severity correlates and comparisons with non-psychiatric controls. *Psychiatry Research* 37, 219-27.

Murphy E (1983) The prognosis depression in old age. *British Journal of Psychiatry* 142, 111-19.

Musetti L, Perugi G, Soriani A et al. (1989) Depression before and after 65. *British Journal of Psychiatry* 155, 330-6.

Oxman TE, Barrett JE, Barrett J and Gerber P (1990) Symptomatology of late-life minor depression among primary care patients. *Psychosomatics* 31, 174-80.

Paykel ES, Prusoff B and Klerman GL (1971) The endogenous-neurotic continuum in depression: rater independence and factor distributions. *Journal of Psychiatric Research* 8, 73-90.

Post F (1972) The management and nature of depressive illness in late life: a follow-through study. *British Journal of Psychiatry* 21, 393-404.

Rovner BW, Broadhead J, Spencer M et al. (1989) Depression and Alzheimer's disease. *American Journal of Psychiatry* 146, 350-3.

Sackeim HA, Freeman J, McElhiney M et al. (1992) Effects of major depression on estimates of intelligence. *Experimental Neuropsychology* 14, 268-88.

Shulman K (1989) Conceptual problems in the assessment of depression in old age. *Psychiatric Journal of the University of Ottawa* 14, 364-71.

Spitzer RL and Endicott J (1978) *Research Diagnostic Criteria for a Selected Group of Functional Disorders* (3rd edn). New York, New York State Psychiatric Institute.

Wragg RE and Jeste DV (1989) Overview of depression and psychosis in Alzheimer's disease. *American Journal of Psychiatry* 146, 577-86.

Zisook S, Shuchter SR and Lyons LE (1987) Predictors of psychological reactions during the early stages of widowhood. *Psychiatric Clinics of North America* 10, 355-68.

2 The Measurement of Depression in Old Age

The detection and measurement of depression in old age is problematic. Under-detection of depression in old age is clinically important, particularly in the primary care context. Though Macdonald (1986) found that general practitioners were able to detect over 90% of elderly surgery attenders with interview-identified depression, much lower detection rates were reported both by Bowers et al. (1990) and Iliffe et al. (1991), who found that GPs miss the overwhelming majority of the cases of (potentially treatable) depression identified by psychiatric interview.

There is thus a clear need for appropriate instruments to detect depression in old age, and to measure its severity. A wide variety of rating scales and interviews, some of them for general adult use and some specific for the elderly, have been used. The merits and disadvantages of the most important of these will be reviewed below. Several considerations must be applied in any such evaluation; these are reviewed succinctly by Applegate (1987). In particular, both validity (the degree to which a measure reflects what it is intended to assess) and reliability (the degree to which repeated measures are consistent) must be considered. Validity may be assessed in terms of correlation with an established instrument (convergent validity) or with clinicians' judgement (criterion validity). If an instrument is designed to detect the presence or absence of depression, its validity can further be estimated in terms of sensitivity (the extent to which depressed patients are identified) and specificity (the extent to which only depressed patients are so classified). Reliability is important in terms both of stability over time (test–retest) and between different practitioners (inter-rater). Choice of instruments needs also to be dictated by the purpose of the investigation. One may wish to make a formal psychiatric diagnosis or simply to screen a population to identify those with a high likelihood of depression. In those patients identified as depressed one may further need to assess initial severity and/or to measure change over time with or without treatment.

Particular problems in measuring depression in old age include an overlap in symptoms with normal elderly subjects, particularly in terms of increases with age in somatic symptoms and insomnia. These issues are discussed in detail in Chapter 1. Kivela and Pahkala (1988a) for example, found that several depressive symptoms conventionally considered indicative of depression, including sleep disturbance, fatiguability, loss of interest, loss of activity, pessimism and a sense of uselessness, were relatively common in non-depressed elderly subjects.

INTERVIEW SCHEDULES

The criterion validity of standard adult diagnostic interviews in the elderly has in general not been assessed. In contrast, the Geriatric Mental Status Schedule (GMS; Copeland et al. 1976) has been designed specifically for psychiatric assessment and diagnosis in an elderly population and has been extensively validated. The GMS was derived from the Present State Examination (PSE; Wing et al. 1974) and the Mental Status Schedule (MSS; Spitzer et al. 1964). The GMS consists of 541 ratings (268 from the PSE, 64 from the MSS and 209 added specifically for use in older subjects). Factor analysis of these ratings generated 21 factors including a depression factor with a total of 51 items comprehensively covering mood, vegetative symptoms, guilt and self-depreciation, interest and concentration. A computerised diagnostic algorithm (AGECAT, Copeland et al. 1986) allows rapid analysis from symptoms through symptom groups and syndrome clusters to diagnoses and severity ratings. The GMS diagnosis of depression shows high criterion validity (88% agreement with clinical diagnosis) and inter-rater reliability ($x = 0.8$) in psychiatric patients with a variety of diagnoses. In a series of epidemiological studies using the GMS in community samples of elderly subjects in New York and London (Copeland et al. 1987b), Liverpool (Copeland et al. 1987a) and Tasmania (Kay et al. 1985), the prevalence of depression was found to be remarkably consistent. The GMS interview and the AGECAT programme are currently available as a software package suitable for use on a laptop computer in field surveys.

Gurland et al. (1977), who were also involved in the development of the GMS, have in parallel developed an assessment schedule for elderly subjects covering physical illness and functional ability as well as psychiatric morbidity. The Comprehensive Assessment and Referral Evaluation (CARE) takes an average of 90 minutes to complete: about one-third of its ratings concern psychiatric problem areas. The psychiatric component of the CARE overlaps very considerably with that of the GMS and has similarly satisfactory inter-rater reliability. A short version of the CARE with depression and cognitive scales but still requiring interview by a trained rater, the SHORT-CARE, has been devised (Gurland et al. 1984). This has been found to be very acceptable in a primary care setting with 100% response rate and high criterion validity against clinical judgement. The depression rating within the SHORT-CARE consists of a total of 18 items and the complete interview takes approximately 15 minutes to perform.

The CAMDEX (Roth et al. 1986) is a relatively new diagnostic interview specific for the elderly which focuses on the detection of early dementia and the distinction between Alzheimer's disease and vascular dementia. It does, however, also include a 20-item depression scale based on interview with the patient and a single question addressed to an informant asking whether the informant considers the patient to be depressed. The CAMDEX depression scale discriminates reasonably well between demented and depressed patients, though not surprisingly there is some overlap, particularly between vascular dementia and depression. It clearly deserves further evaluation as a screening and diagnostic instrument.

INTERVIEW-BASED RATING SCALES

A number of interview-based rating scales for depression initially developed for younger adults have been used in studies of elderly patients. The most popular of these has been the Hamilton Depression Rating Scale (HDRS; Hamilton 1967). As discussed in Chapter 3, Kivela and Pahkala (1988b) carried out a factor analysis of HDRS items. Though the first of these factors was similar to the general depression factor found in a younger population by Hamilton (1967), the second factor identified by Hamilton (corresponding to the unipolar/bipolar distinction), was only found in depressed elderly men. The HDRS thus clearly behaves differently in older subjects. It should also be noted that the HDRS was not designed for screening but for evaluating severity and typology of depression in those for whom the diagnosis of depression had already been made. Furthermore, the HDRS is relatively heavily weighted for items measuring somatic symptomatology and sleep disturbance, which reduce its face validity in an elderly population. The Montgomery–Asberg Depression Rating Scale (MADRS; Montgomery and Asberg 1979) is also widely used for interview-based evaluation in younger depressed patients. Sleep, anxiety and somatic items are given less weighting than in the HDRS, and the MADRS was designed specifically to be sensitive to change. It is also more appropriate as a general screening instrument (prior to a formal diagnosis of depression being made) since it forms part of a larger psychiatric screening interview, the Comprehensive Psychopathological Rating Scale (Asberg et al. 1978). Agrell and Dehlin (1989), in a study of geriatric stroke patients, found the MADRS to have excellent criterion validity ($r = 0.86$) against a global clinical rating of depression as well as showing satisfactory internal consistency and high sensitivity (88%) and specificity (70%). It has not, however, had formal criterion validation in a community elderly population.

Blazer (1980) has devised a brief interview-based rating specifically for use in the elderly, the OARS Depressive Scale (ODS). Factor analysis of the ODS in depressed subjects generated three factors: dysphoric mood, depressive diagnosis and pessimism. Together, these explained 87% of the total scale variance. The ODS shows good criterion validity, with agreement in 90% of inpatient and 75% of community subjects. Though influential in identifying a significant group of elderly subjects with dysphoric mood but not fulfilling DSM III major depression criteria, the ODS has not subsequently been widely used.

SUBJECT-COMPLETED RATING SCALES

Subject-completed rating scales, though not specifically designed for such use, have none the less been widely applied in the elderly. They include the Centre for Epidemiological Studies in Depression Scale (CES-D; Murrell et al. 1983), the Self-rating Depression Scale (SDS; Zung 1965) and the Beck Scale (Beck et al. 1961).

The CES-D, though used in a very large epidemiological study (Murrell et al. 1983), was able to identify only 70% of the depressed subjects in an elderly inpatient population and found 14% of a community sample to score above the depression cut-off point. The SDS has been shown (Reforge and Sogal 1988) to correspond closely (88% agreement) with the CES-D; the CES-D, however, identified many more subjects as depressed than the SDS. The authors considered that this reflected the relative preponderance of psychological items in the CES-D and somatic ones in the SDS. Most subjects in the study suffered from osteoarthritis and no criterion validation against clinician diagnosis was attempted.

A self-completed rating scale specifically for elderly subjects, the Geriatric Depression Scale (GDS; see the Appendix at the end of this chapter), which can also be completed through interview, has been devised by Yesavage et al. (1983). The GDS consists of 30 Yes/No items. In their original report, Yesavage et al. (1983) showed the GDS to have highly satisfactory consistency ($\alpha = 0.94$), split-half reliability ($r = 0.94$), and test–retest reliability ($r = 0.85$). The GDS has been validated against Research Diagnostic Criteria (RDC; Spitzer and Endicott 1978) diagnoses and its performance compared with the SDS and the HDRS. The GDS performed better than either of the other scales in terms of sensitivity and specificity (specificity 80%, sensitivity 90%) and correlated highly with both. It performed as well as the HDRS, and significantly better than the SDS, in distinguishing between normal, mildly depressed and severely depressed subjects on RDC criteria. The GDS has been validated against the GMS interview in a British primary care sample of elderly patients by Evans and Katona (1993). It showed satisfactory sensitivity (85%) and specificity (68%), and agreed significantly more often (76% vs 65) with GMS diagnosis than did GPs' own assessments.

The GDS has recently been validated in both Italian and Spanish translation. Mardi et al. (1991) found that the standard cut-off of 10/11 yielded a sensitivity of 91% and a specificity of 91% against the DSM IIIR spectrum of depressive disorders. Similarly high sensitivity (94%) and specificity (94%) have been reported by Brieva et al. (1991), though with a substantially higher cut-off (16/17). This study also reported a very satisfactory overall level of agreement ($x = 0.88$) for case/non-case against 'hospital criteria' for depression. Satisfactory longitudinal stability of the GDS has been established in the original validation sample ($r = 0.94$), and in a group of frail nursing home residents ($r = 0.82$) by Abraham (1991).

A short (15-item) version of the GDS (GDS–15) has been devised by Sheikh and Yesavage (1986), taking only 5–7 minutes to administer and with the aim of achieving greater client acceptability. This scale (see the Appendix at the end of this chapter), consisting of the items from the original scale showing highest correlation with depressive symptoms, has been reported to correlate significantly ($r = 0.66$) with the parent scale (Alden et al. 1989). With a cut-off of 6/7, it has also been found (Burke et al. 1991) to have similar sensitivity in cognitively intact elderly subjects (78%), but somewhat lower specificity (67%). The same study found that a lower cut-off (4/5) gave a specificity of only 48% but identified 93% of depressed subjects. Katona et al. (1994) have recently used logistic regression analysis to derive a four-item version of the GDS which had a specificity of up to 88% (cut-off 1/2) and sensitivity of up to 93% (cut-off 0/1) against the GMS interview. This version (shown as the items in bold on the 15-item GDS reproduced in the Appendix), though in need of further testing, may be useful as a 'first level' screen in primary care.

The GDS thus appears to represent a considerable advance in providing acceptable and valid screening for depression in elderly subjects. It also provides a validated measure of severity: scores of 0–10 being regarded as not depressed, 11–20 as mild depression and >20 as severe depression.

Patient compliance with the GDS (15-item version) administered as a short interview to a primary care sample was found to be very high by D'Ath et al. (1994). Ninety-eight per cent completed the interview and only 13% found it difficult, stressful or unacceptable. It should be noted that, in elderly subjects, interviews may be associated with higher completion rates than questionnaires. Toner et al. (1988) found that whereas a self-administered questionnaire (in their case the SDS) was frequently not filled in satisfactorily, a brief interview (the SHORT-CARE) was invariably completed successfully. Although the GDS may be administered either for self-rating or by interview it has yet to be established whether the scale performs identically with these different methods of administration.

Two self-completed versions of the depression scale from the SHORT-CARE (Gurland et al. 1984) have been devised and subjected to preliminary testing as screening instruments. Both are reproduced in the Appendix at the end of this chapter. The first, the SELFCARE-D (Bird et al. 1987), consists of 12 questions, each with choices of answer graded by severity of symptom. The SELFCARE-D was found at initial testing to have a sensitivity of 77% and specificity of 98% ($x = 0.77$) against the clinical diagnosis made by a research psychiatrist in a sample of 75 elderly primary care attenders. It also appeared to perform better than the SDS, though formal comparison results are not reported. The second, the Brief Assessment Schedule Depression Cards (BASDEC; Adshead et al. 1992) consists of 19 cards, each representing items from the SHORT-CARE and to be answered as 'true' or 'false'. BASDEC represents a hybrid between self-completed and interview-based screening instruments. It was tested in a sample of 79 elderly medical inpatients in terms both of convergent validity (against the GDS) and criterion validity (against a research psychiatrist's clinical diagnosis). More patients completed the BASDEC than the GDS, suggesting that the BASDEC is highly acceptable. Agreement between the scales occurred in 87% of cases, with both scales having identical sensitivity (71%) and specificity (88%) against clinical diagnosis. Both SELFCARE-D and BASDEC represent potentially useful alternatives to the GDS and clearly warrant further field testing.

The specific problem of screening for suicide risk in an elderly depressed population has been addressed by Hill et al. (1988) who assessed the performance of the Hopelessness Scale of Beck et al. (1974b). Not only did the scale have satisfactory internal consistency and a factor structure similar to that found in the original younger validation sample, but it correlated significantly with suicidality as measured by clinical interview. It should be noted, however, that the scale accounted for only 27% of the variance of clinically assessed suicidality and has not been validated in an elderly population in terms of ability to predict subsequent suicidal behaviour. A related scale, the Beck Suicidal Intent Scale (Beck et al. 1974a) has been subjected to more stringent validation by Pierce (1987), who administered it to a consecutive group of elderly cases of deliberate self-harm, and found highly significant differences in scores between those who subsequently killed themselves and those who did not.

MEASURING DEPRESSION IN PHYSICALLY ILL AND/OR DEMENTED SUBJECTS

The studies outlined above have addressed the issue of interview and rating scale validity in elderly subjects drawn from community and primary care populations. A new range of problems emerges in the large subgroups of elderly subjects with coexistent physical illness and/or cognitive impairment. Detection of depression in physically ill or demented elderly subjects may be importantsince such depression symptomatology may be amenable to treatment and, in the case of physically ill subjects may worsen the prognosis of the physical condition.

Koenig et al. (1988) found that medically ill patients with major depression consumed more health care resources as well as experiencing greater mortality than their non-depressed counterparts. Coexistent depression may also prolong length of hospital stay in the physically ill elderly (Gurland et al. 1988).

The detection of depression in elderly physically ill subjects is notoriously difficult. Rapp et al. (1988) found that only 8.7% of depressed patients admitted with physical illness were identified by house staff. A similar low rate of documentation of depressive symptoms by house staff (20%) was reported by Koenig et al. (1988) which only increased to 27% after they had been informed of the possibility of major depression. The GMS interview also performs quite poorly in elderly physically ill subjects (Copeland et al. 1986), in particular showing low inter-rater reliability ($x = 50\%$).

In contrast, Rapp et al. (1988), who compared the performance of the SDS, Beck and GDS in acute elderly medical admissions, found that both the Beck and the GDS showed satisfactory criterion validity against RDC. An earlier study (Okimoto et al. 1982), using the SDS, found that although it correctly identified

80% of elderly medical patients with DSM III major depression, much higher sensitivity and specificity was achieved using a brief six-item scale devoid of somatic items. A similar study of the Beck scale (Cavanaugh et al. 1983) compared healthy elderly, depressed elderly and medically ill elderly subjects. The overall sensitivity and specificity of the Beck Scale in detecting major depression in the physically ill was not reported, but a subscale involving seven items (feeling like a failure, loss of interest in people, feeling punished, suicidal ideation, dissatisfaction, difficulty with decisions and crying) best discriminated depressive severity in the three groups.

Lyons et al. (1989) have shown that the GDS is test–retest and inter-rater reliable, internally consistent and highly correlated with the HDRS in elderly patients with hip fracture. Similar findings in geriatric stroke patients have been reported by Agrell and Dehlin (1989), who found the GDS to show a correlation of 0.75 against a global rating of depression and to have a sensitivity of 88% and specificity of 64% in detecting depression in such patients. Ramsay et al. (1991) have demonstrated that the GDS has satisfactory sensitivity (74%) and specificity (72%) against the SHORT-CARE depression scale in detecting significant depressive symptomatology in acute elderly medical admissions. All cases of full-blown depressive illness were detected, but the specificity of the GDS for depressive illness was only 50%. Harper et al. (1990), however, found that the GDS failed to identify 15% of elderly medically ill patients with RDC major depression and as many as 58% of those with minor depression. The GDS may also perform less well in subjects with chronic physical illness partly because of a relatively high rate of cognitive impairment. Kafonek et al. (1989) evaluated the GDS in a long-term care facility and found it to have satisfactory specificity (75%) but low sensitivity (47%) in this population. The poor performance of the GDS in this study was attributable entirely to a sensitivity of only 25% in the cognitively impaired subgroup. Shah et al. (1992), however, found that with the same optimal cut-off point (12/13) as used by Harper et al. (1990), the GDS showed sensitivity of 75% and specificity of 73% in a cohort of patients in continuing care geriatric beds.

The detection of depression within dementia is also problematic. Depression within Alzheimer's disease is particularly difficult to measure. This is partly because of the lack of an adequate 'gold standard'. As Christensen and Dyksen (1990) have pointed out, DSM IIIR criteria for depression may be very misleading in demented patients since so many of the depression items are also found in nondepressed subjects with Alzheimer's disease—the most obvious example of this being diminished ability to think or concentrate. Several studies, reviewed by Wragg and Jeste (1989), have none the less confirmed that significant depressive symptomatology frequently occurs in dementia. Such depression is apparently worth treating: a double-blind trial comparing imipramine with placebo (Reifler et al. 1989) found that moderate depression in patients with Alzheimer's disease responded significantly to active treatment.

Several approaches to the problem of measurement have been adopted. Some studies have, despite the problems outlined above, used checklists based on DSM

III or DSM IIIR criteria (Reifler et al. 1982; Rovner et al. 1989). Others have used standard adult depression rating scales like the HDRS (Lazarus et al. 1987). Burke et al. (1989) have attempted to validate the GDS in a sample of patients with dementia of the Alzheimer type using clinical diagnoses as the standard for criterion validation. In their study the GDS discriminated less well between depressed and non-depressed subjects in the presence of Alzheimer's disease than in its absence; indeed, in the demented patients there was no cut-off point at which the GDS discriminated for depression better than chance alone. They have also reported similar performance (again no better than chance) for the GDS–15 in cognitively impaired subjects (Burke et al. 1991). This is in keeping with the findings of Kafonek et al. (1989) but contrasts with Shah et al. (1992), who reported satisfactory performance for the GDS, using a modified cut-off of 12/13, in the demented subsample of a group of elderly physically ill subjects in continuing care.

It is clear from the above that the applicability of more generally useful diagnostic systems and rating scales for measuring depression in demented subjects may be limited. An important reason for this may be that demented patients consistently underestimate their own depression rather than giving random responses. MacKenzie et al. (1989) compared data elicited from demented patients themselves and from their families in completing checklists of DSM III major depression items. Depression was found in only 14% of the subjects when the diagnosis was derived from their own responses, whereas information from their families indicated a rate of 50%. Family reports exceeded those of patients themselves most markedly in reporting loss of interest, irritability, fatigue and worthlessness.

In view of these difficulties, a number of scales have been developed specifically designed to detect depression in demented subjects. These rely more or less exclusively on items rated objectively by the interviewer or on information about patient behaviour gleaned from an observer. The NIMH Dementia Mood Assessment Scale (DMAS; Sunderland et al. 1988) has 17 items measuring depression, including depressed appearance such as and physical agitation as well as more subjective ones like guilt feelings and self-esteem. The authors report the scale to have satisfactory inter-rater reliability and to correlate significantly ($r = 0.73$) with a global measure of depression, and with the HDRS ($r = 0.47$). The Cornell Scale for Depression in Dementia (Alexopoulos et al. 1988) is quite similar, showing high inter-rater reliability ($\varkappa = 0.67$) and consistency ($\alpha = 0.84$), as well as correlating significantly ($r = 0.83$) with severity of depression as measured by RDC criteria, and more weakly ($r = 0.54$) with HDRS score. The Cornell Scale also appears sensitive to change in hospitalised dementia subjects with major depression improving with treatment. Both these scales remain reliant on subjective items. The DMAS has been validated only in patients with mild to moderate dementia. The Cornell Scale appeared in its original validation study (Alexopoulos et al. 1988) to retain inter-rater reliability and to correlate with RDC depression ratings (but not with HDRS scores) in more severely demented subjects, but was found by Agrell and Dehlin (1989) to show poor validity in geriatric stroke patients.

The Depressive Signs Scale (DSS; Katona and Aldridge 1985) is a much shorter scale consisting of nine items focusing entirely on observed behaviour. It has been subjected to less exhaustive validation but has satisfactory inter-rater reliability. Within demented subjects, high scorers were significantly more likely to show dexamethasone suppression test non-suppression. The DSS has has recently (Katona et al. 1992) been shown to discriminate significantly between depressed, demented and healthy elderly subjects, though DSS scores did not (in keeping with the findings using the Cornell Scale in a severely demented sample) show significant correlation with the HDRS. Subjects with dementia showed a much wider scatter of scores than either healthy or depressed subjects.

The use of one of these dementia-specific scales is to be strongly recommended in evaluating demented patients whose depressive symptoms, although clinically relevant, may not otherwise be detected. These scales have not, however, been validated in the clinically important exercise of distinguishing dementia complicated by depression from depressive pseudodementia.

CONCLUSIONS: THE UTILITY OF CASE DETECTION INSTRUMENTS

There are as yet no ideal instruments for measuring depression in old age, but the many instruments designed specifically for this purpose represent a major step forward from those designed for use in younger adults. Choice of instrument depends crucially on the use to which any data collected is to be put. The 'best-available' options for a variety of uses are summarised in Table 2.1. The GMS has been extensively used to good effect to resolve apparent epidemiological incon-sistency (see Chapter 3) and its portable computer version renders it still more attractive for further epidemiological use. The GDS is now widely used as an acceptable screening instrument, and has recently been endorsed (in its 15-item version) as the appropriate screening instrument for statutory health checks in primary care patients aged 75 and over (Williams and Wallace 1993). Among instruments not specifically designed for use in the elderly, the MADRS is probably the best choice for screening.

There is as yet no ideal solution to the problem of detecting depression in elderly subjects with coexistent physical illness and/or dementia. The currently available scales for measuring depression within established dementia are a step in the right direction but require further validation and (probably) modification. No specific scale for measuring depression in the physically ill has yet been fully validated, though preliminary data on such a scale (which makes use of nursing observations as well as items elicited directly from patients) have been reported by Evans (1993). Such a scale would be a major contribution to the liaison psychiatry of old age. Meanwhile, most studies suggest that the GDS remains

Table 2.1   Appropriate case detection instruments

Purpose	Appropriate instrument(s)
Research diagnosis	GMS
	CAMDEX
Primary care screening	GDS-15
	SELFCARE-D
Primary care diagnosis	SHORT-CARE
Residential care screening	GDS-30
	SELFCARE-D
	Cornell Scale
	DMAS
	DSS
Residential care diagnosis	SHORT-CARE
Geriatric medicine screening	GDS-30
	SELFCARE-D
	BASDEC
Geriatric medicine diagnosis	SHORT-CARE

useful in physically ill patients. Though less extensively evaluated, BASDEC may be an acceptable alternative. The GDS has recently been recommended as the best available screening test (the SDS, SELFCARE-D and HDRS having also been considered) for depression in the context of geriatric medicine by the Royal College of Physicians of London and the British Geriatrics Society (Royal College of Physicians and British Geriatrics Society 1992).

REFERENCES

Abraham IL (1991) The Geriatric Depression Scale and Hopelessness Index: longitudinal psychometric data on frail nursing home residents. *Perceptual and Motor Skills* 72, 875–80.
Adshead F, Cody DD and Pitt B (1992) BASDEC: a novel screening instrument for depression in elderly medical patients. *British Medical Journal* 305, 397.
Agrell B and Dehlin O (1989) Comparison of six depression rating scales in geriatric stroke patients. *Stroke* 60, 1190–4.
Alden D, Austin C and Sturgeon R (1989) A correlation between the Geriatric Depression Scale long and shout forms. *Journal of Gerontology: Psychological Sciences* 44, 124–5.
Alexopoulos GS, Abrams RC, Young RC and Shamoian CA (1988) Cornell Scale for Depression in Dementia. *Biological Psychiatry* 23, 271–84.
Applegate WB (1987) Use of assessment instruments in clinical settings. *Journal of the American Geriatric Society* 35, 45–50.
Asberg M, Montgomery SA, Perris C et al. (1978) A comprehensive psychopathological rating scale. *Acta Psychiatrica Scandinavica* Suppl. 271, 5–27.

Beck AT, Schuyler D and Herman J (1974a) Development of suicidal intent scales. In Beck AT, Resnick L and Lettieri BBG (eds) *Prediction of Suicide*. Maryland, Charles Press.

Beck AT, Ward CH, Mendelson M et al. (1961) An inventory for measuring depression. *Archives of General Psychiatry* 4, 561–71.

Beck AT, Weissman A, Lester D and Trexler L (1974b) The measurement of pessimism: the Hopelessness Scale. *Journal of Consulting and Clinical Psychology* 42, 861–5.

Bird AS, Macdonald AJD, Mann AH, Philpot MP (1987) Preliminary experience with the SELF CARE D. *International Journal of Geriatric Psychiatry* 2, 31–8.

Blazer D (1980) The diagnosis of depression in he elderly. *Journal of the American Geriatric Society* 28, 52–8.

Bowers J, Jorm AF, Henderson S and Harris P (1990) General practitioners' detection of depression and demetia in elderly patients. *Medical Journal of Australia* 153, 192–196.

Brieva JAR, Iglesias MLM, Lopez RL et al. (1991) Validacion de la escala-scriba geriatrica para la depresion. *Actas Luso-Espanolas Neurologia y Psiquiatria* 3, 174–7.

Burke WJ, Houston MJ, Boust SJ and Roccaforte WH (1989) Use of the Geriatric Depression Scale in dementia of the Alzheimer type. *Journal of the American Geriatric Society* 37, 856–60.

Burke WJ, Roccaforte WH and Wengel SP (1991) The short form of the Geriatric Depression Scale: a comparison with the 30-item form. *Journal of Geriatric Psychiatry and Neurology* 4, 173–8.

Cavanaugh S, Clark DC and Gibbons RD (1983) Diagnosing depression in the hospitalised medically ill. *Psychosomatics* 24, 809–15.

Christensen KJ and Dyksen MW (1990) The Geriatric Depression Scale in Alzheimer's disease. *Journal of the American Geriatric Society* 38, 724–5.

Copeland JRM, Kelleher MJ, Kellett JM and Gourlay AJ (1976) A semi-structured clinical interview for the assessment of diagnosis and mental state in the elderly: the Geriatric Mental State Schedule. *Psychological Medicine* 6, 439–49.

Copeland JRM, Dewey ME and Griffiths-Jones HM (1986) A computerised psychiatric diagnostic system and case nomenclature for elderly subjects: GMS and AGECAT. *Psychological Medicine* 16, 89–99.

Copeland JRM, Gurland BJ, Dewey ME et al. (1987b) Is there more dementia, depression and neurosis in New York? A comparative community study of the elderly in New York and London using the community diagnosis AGECAT. *British Journal of Psychiatry* 151, 466–73.

Copeland JRM, Dewey ME, Wood N et al. (1987a) Range of mental illness among the elderly in the community: prevalence in Liverpool using the GMS-AGECAT package. *British Journal of Psychiatry* 150, 815–23.

D'Ath P, Katona P, Mullan E and Katona CLE (1994) The acceptability and performance of the 15-item Geriatric Depression Scale (GDS15) in elderly primary care attenders. Submitted for publication.

DeForge BR and Sobal J (1988) Self-report depression scales in the elderly: the relationship between the CES-D and Zung. *International Journal of Psychiatry in Medicine* 18, 325–38.

Evans M (1993) Development and validation of a brief screening scale for depression in the elderly physically ill. In *Advances in Old Age Psychiatry*, pp. 15–16. Abingdon, The Medicine Group.

Evans S and Katona CLE (1993) Depressive symptoms in elderly primary care attenders. *Dementia*, in press.

Gurland B, Golden RR, Teresi JA and Challop J (1984) The SHORT-CARE: an efficient instrument for the assessment of depession, dementia and disability. *Journal of Gerontology* 39, 166–9.

Gurland B, Kuriansky J, Sharpe L et al. (1977) The Comprehensive Assessment and Referral Evaluation (CARE)—Rationale development and reliability. *International Journal of Aging and Human Development* **8**, 9–42.

Gurland BJ, Wilder DE, Golden R et al. (1988) The relationship between depression and disability in the elderly—data from the comprehensive assessment and referral evaluation (CARE). In Wattis JP and Hindmarch I (eds) *Psychological Assessment of the Elderly*. Edinburgh, Churchill Livingstone,

Hamilton M (1967) Development of a rating scale for primary depressive illnes. *British Journal of Social and Clinical Psychology* **6**, 278–96.

Harper RG, Kotik-Harper D and Kirby H. (1990) Psychometric assessment of depression in an elderly general medical population. *Journal of Nervous and Mental Diseases* **178**, 113–19.

Hill RD, Gallagher D, Thompson LW and Ishida T (1988) Hopelessness as a measure of suicidal intent in the depressed elderly. *Psychology and Aging* **3**, 230–2.

Iliffe S, Haines A, Gallivan S et al. (1991) Assessment of elderly people in general practice 1. Social circumstances and mental state. *British Journal of General Practice* **41**, 9–12.

Kafonek S, Ettinger WH, Roca R et al. (1989) Instruments for screening for depression and dementia in a long-term care facility. *Journal of the American Geriatric Society* **37**, 29–34.

Katona CLE and Aldridge CR (1985) The dexamethasone suppression test and depressive signs in dementia. *Journal of Affective Disorders* **8**, 83–9.

Katona CLE, Evans S, D'Ath P et al. (1994) The development of short screening instruments for detecting depression in elderly primary care patients. Submitted for publication.

Katona CLE, Mullan M and Taylor C (1992) Depressive disorders and organic brain disorders: validation of the Depressive Signs Scale. *Clinical Neuropharmacology* **15**, 281A–2A.

Kay DWK, Henderson AS, Scott R et al. (1985) Dementia and depression among the elderly living in the Hobart community: the effect of diagnostic criteria on the prevalence rates. *Pschological Medicine* **15**, 771–8.

Kivela S-L and Pahkala K (1988a) Clinician-rated symptoms and signs of depression in aged Finns. *International Journal of Social Psychiatry* **34**, 274–84.

Kivela S-L and Pahkala K (1988b) Factor structure of the Hamilton rating scale for depression among depressed elderly Finns. *Zeitschrift für Psychologie* **196**, 389–99.

Koenig HG, Meador KG, Cohen HJ and Blazer DG (1988) Detection and treatment of major depression in older medically ill hospitalised patients. *International Journal of Psychiatry in Medicine* **18**, 17–31.

Lazarus LW, Newton N, Cohler B et al. (1987) Frequency and presentation of depressive symptoms in patients with primary degenerative dementia. *American Journal of Psychiatry* **144**, 41–5.

Lyons JS, Strain JJ, Hammer JS et al. (1989) Reliability, validity and temporal stability of the Geriatric Depression Scale in hospitalised elderly. *International Journal of Psychiatry in Medicine* **19**, 203–9.

Macdonald AJP (1986) Do general practitioners 'miss' depression in elderly patients? *British Medical Journal* **292**, 365–7.

Mackenzie TB, Robiner WN and Knopman DS (1989) Differences between patient and family assessments of depression in Alzheimer's disease. *American Journal of Psychiatry* **146**, 1174–8.

Montgomery SA and Asberg M (1979) A new depression scale designed to be sensitive to change. *British Journal of Psychiatry* **134**, 382–9.

Murrell SA, Himmelfarb S and Wright K (1983) Prevalence of depression and its correlates in older adults. *American Journal of Epidemiology* **117**, 173–85.

Nardi B, de Rosa M, Paciaroni G et al. (1991) Indagine clinica sulla depressione in un campione randomizzato e stratificato di popolazione anziana. *Minerva Psychiatrica* **32**, 135–44.

Okimoto JT, Barnes RF, Veith RC et al. (1982) Screening for depression in geriatric medical patients. *American Journal of Psychiatry* **136**, 799–802.

Pierce D (1987) Deliberate self-harm in the elderly. *International Journal of Geriatric Psychiatry* **2**, 105–10.

Ramsay R, Wright P, Katz A et al. (1991) The detection of psychiatric morbidity and its effects on outcome in acute elderly medical admissions. *International Journal of Geriatric Psychiatry* **6**, 861–6.

Rapp SR, Walsh DA, Parisi SA and Wallace CE (1988) Detecting depression in elderly medical inpatients. *Journal of Consulting and Clinical Psychology* **56**, 509–13.

Reifler BV, Larson E and Handley R (1982) Coexistence of cognitive impairment and depression in geriatric outpatients. *American Journal of Psychiatry* **139**, 623–6.

Reifler BV, Teri L, Raskind M et al. (1989) Double-blind trial of imipramine in Alzheimer's disease patients with and without depression. *American Journal of Psychiatry* **146**, 45–9.

Roth M, Tym E, Mountjoy CQ et al. (1986) CAMDEX: a standardised instrument for the diagnosis of mental disorder in the elderly with special reference to the early detection of dementia. *British Journal of Psychiatry* **149**, 698–709.

Rover BW, Broadhead J, Spencer M et al. (1989) Depression and Alzheimer's Disease. *American Journal of Psychiatry* **146**, 350–3.

Royal College of Physicians and British Geriatrics Society (1992) *Standardised Assessment Scales for Elderly People*. Report of Joint Workshops of the Research Unit of the Royal College of Physicians and the British Geriatrics Society. London, Royal College of Physicians.

Shah A, Phongsathorn V, George C et al. (1992) Psychiatric morbidity among continuing care geriatric in-patients. *International Journal of Geriatric Psychiatry* **7**, 517–25.

Sheikh JA and Yesavage JA (1986) Geriatric Depression Scale (GDS): recent findings and development of a shorter version. In Brink TL (ed.) Clinical Gerontology: A Guide to Assessment and Intervention. New York, Howarth Press.

Spitzer RL and Endicott J (1978) *Research Diagnostic Criteria for a Selected Group of Functional Disorders* (3rd edn). New York, New York State Psychiatric Institute.

Spitzer RL, Fleiss JL, Burdock EI and Hardesty AS (1964) The mental status schedule: rationale, reliability and validity. *Comprehensive Psychiatry* **5**, 384–95.

Sunderland T, Hill JL, Lawlor BA and Molchan SE (1988) NIMH Dementia Mood Asessment Scale (DMAS). *Psychopharmacology Bulletin* **24**, 747–9.

Toner J, Burland B and Teresi J. (1988) Comparison of self-administered and rater-administered methods of assessing levels of severity of depression in elderly patients. *Journal of Gerontology* **43**, 136–40.

Williams EI and Wallace P (1993) Health checks for people aged 75 and over. British Journal of General Practice Occasional Paper No. 59.

Wing JK, Cooper JE and Sartorius N (1974) *The Measurement and Classification of Psychiatric Symptoms*. Cambridge, Cambridge University Press.

Wragg RE and Jeste DV (1989) Overview of depression and psychosis in Alzheimer's disease. *American Journal of Psychiatry* **146**, 577–86.

Yesavage JA, Brink TL, Rose TL and Lum O (1983) Development and validation of a geriatric depression screening scale: a preliminary report. *Journal of Psychiatric Research* **17**, 37–49.

Zung WWK (1965) A self-rating depression scale. *Archives of General Psychiatry* **12**, 63–70.

Appendix

The main instruments specifically designed to screen for depression in old age (GDS-30, GDS-15, SELFCARE-D, BASDEC) are reproduced below.

THE GERIATRIC DEPRESSION SCALE*

30-ITEM VERSION (GDS-30)

Are you basically-satisfied with your life?	Yes/NO
Have you dropped many of your activities and interests?	YES/No
Do you feel that your life is empty?	YES/No
Do you often get bored?	YES/No
Are you hopeful about the future?	Yes/NO
Are you bothered by thoughts you can't get out of your head?	YES/No
Are you in good spirits most of the time?	Yes/NO
Are you afraid that something bad is going to happen to you?	YES/No
Do you feel happy most of the time?	Yes/NO
Do you often feel helpless?	YES/No
Do you often get restless and fidgety?	YES/No
Do you prefer to stay at home, rather than going out and doing new things?	YES/No
Do you frequently worry about the future?	YES/No
Do you feel you have more problems with memory than most?	YES/No
Do you think it is wonderful to be alive now?	Yes/NO
Do you often feel downhearted and blue?	YES/No
Do you feel pretty worthless the way you are now?	YES/No
Do you worry a lot about the past?	YES/No
Do you find life very exciting?	Yes/NO
Is it hard for you to get started on new projects?	YES/No
Do you feel full of energy?	Yes/NO
Do you feel that your situation is hopeless?	YES/No
Do you think that most people are better off than you are?	YES/No
Do you frequently get upset over little things?	YES/No
Do you frequently feel like crying?	YES/No
Do you have trouble concentrating?	YES/No
Do you enjoy getting up in the morning?	Yes/NO
Do you prefer to avoid social gatherings?	YES/No
Is it easy for you to make decisions?	Yes/NO
Is your mind as clear as it used to be?	Yes/NO

Scoring

Score 1 for answer in capitals. 0–10: not depressed; 11–20: mild depression; 21–30: severe depression.

---

*Reproduced from Yesavage et al. (1983) *Journal of Psychiatric Research* 17, 37–49, by kind permission of Pergamon Press Ltd.

15-ITEM VERSION (GDS-16). (4-ITEM GDS SHOWN AS ITEMS IN BOLD)

Are you basically satisfied with your life?	Yes/NO
Have you dropped many of your activities and interests?	YES/No
Do you feel that your life is empty?	YES/No
Do you often get bored?	YES/No
Are you in good spirits most of the time?	Yes/NO
Are you afraid that something bad is going to happen to you?	YES/No
Do you feel happy most of the time?	Yes/NO
Do you often feel helpless?	YES/No
Do you prefer to stay at home, rather than going out and doing new things?	YES/No
Do you feel you have more problems with memory than most?	YES/No
Do you think it is wonderful to be alive now?	Yes/NO
Do you feel pretty worthless the way you are now?	YES/No
Do you feel full of energy?	Yes/NO
Do you feel that your situation is hopeless?	YES/No
Do you think that most people are better off than you are?	YES/No

Scoring

Score 1 for answer in capitals. 0–5: not depressed; 6–15: depressed.
(In 4-item version, score of 0: not depressed; 1: uncertain; >1: probably depressed.)

THE SELFCARE-D*

1 How is your health compared with others of your age?

Excellent
Good
Fair
Don't know what is meant by question

2 How quick in your movements are you-compared with a year ago?

Quicker than usual
About as quick as usual
Less quick than usual
Considerably slower than usual
Don't know what is meant by question

---

*Reproduced from Bird et al. (1987), *International Journal of Geriatric Psychiatry* **2**, 31–38, by permission.

3 How much energy do you have compared with a year ago?

   More than usual
   About the same as usual
   Less than usual
   Hardly any at all
   Don't know what is meant by question

4 In the last month have you had any headaches?

   Not at all
   About the same as usual
   Some of the time
   A lot of the time
   All of the time
   Don't know what is meant by question

5 Have you worried about things this past month?

   Not at all
   Only now and then
   Some of the time
   A lot of the time
   All of the time
   Don't know what is meant by question

6 Have you been sad, unhappy (depressed) or weepy in the past month?

   Not at all
   Only now and then
   Some of the time
   A lot of the time
   All of the time
   Don't know what is meant by question

7 In the past month, have you been lying awake at night feeling uneasy or unhappy?

   Not at all
   Once or twice
   Quite often
   Very often
   Don't know what is meant by question

8 Do you blame yourself for unpleasant things that have happened?

   Not at all
   About one thing
   About a few things
   About everything
   Don't know what is meant by question

9 How do you feel about your future?

Very happy
Quite happy
All right
Unsure
Don't care
Worried
Frightened
Hopeless
Don't know what is meant by question

10 What have you enjoyed doing lately?

Everything
Most things
Some things
One or two things
Nothing
Don't know what is meant by question

11 In the past month, have there been times when you've felt quite happy?

Often
Sometimes
Now and then
Never
Don't know what is meant by question

12 In general, how happy are you?

Very happy
Fairly happy
Not very happy
Not happy at all
Don't know what is meant by question

Scoring

Score 1 for each item in bold. Recommended case/non-case cut-off is 5/6. If 'don't know' option is selected four or more times, scale is unreliable. If this option is selected three times or less, final score can be ascertained on a proportional basis.

BASDEC (BRIEF ASSESSMENT SCHEDULE DEPRESSION CARDS)

Each item in this scale is reproduced on a separate, large-print card. The instructions for its administration are as follows.

1   Remove **TRUE** and **FALSE** cards from pack
2   Shuffle pack of cards
3   Hand the cards, one by one, to the patient
4   Ask the patient to place the cards in one of two piles '**TRUE**' or '**FALSE**'
5   Any cards which cause confusion or doubt should be placed in a 'don't know' pile
    (these may form a useful focal point for discussion)

The cards

I've been depressed for weeks at a time in the past
I am a nuisance to others being ill
I'm not happy at all
I seem to have lost my appetite
I have regrets about my past life
I'm kept awake by worry and unhappy thoughts
I've felt very low lately
I've seriously considered suicide
I feel anxious all the time
I feel life is hardly worth living
I feel worst at the beginning of the day
I'm too miserable to enjoy anything
I'm so lonely
I can't recall feeling happy in the past month
I suffer headaches
I'm not sleeping well
I've lost interest in things
I've cried in the past month
I've given up hope
True
False

Scoring

Each 'TRUE' card has a value of **ONE POINT**. Each '**DON'T KNOW**' card has a value of **HALF A POINT**. The cards in the '**FALSE**' pile do not score. The exceptions to this are the cards
'I've given up hope'
'I've seriously considered suicide'
which have values of **TWO POINTS** if '**TRUE**' and **ONE POINT** if '**DON'T KNOW**'.
   A patient scoring a total of **SEVEN** or more points may well be suffering from a depressive disorder.

Reproduced from Adshead et al. (1992) *British Medical Journal* **305**, 397,© Merck *Pharmaceuticals*.

3 The Epidemiology of Depression in Old Age

Estimates of the prevalence of depression in the elderly vary widely (Post and Shulman 1985). Such discrepancies result from a number of methodological problems that have only recently been adequately addressed.

The first major problem is in the selection of subjects to be studied. This area is well reviewed by Kay and Bergmann (1980), who emphasise that hospital-based samples are particularly highly selected and unrepresentative. They regard tracing a community cohort over time as the ideal method, although seldom practicable; most studies have adopted a 'census' approach, studying a defined population over a short period.

Freedman et al. (1982) suggest family practitioner consultation as an appropriate point, from a clinical as well as a research point of view, for making accurate estimates of depression in the elderly. Not only do the great majority of elderly people see their family practitioner regularly, but the family practitioner's role in the care of the individual's physical and psychological well-being provides the opportunity for making the detection of depression the starting point for its appropriate management.

The definition of depression within the population being studied represents a further problem. Copeland (1981) has made a valuable contribution to our understanding of the concept of a psychiatric 'case', particularly in relation to the question of intervention. Criteria for individual symptoms need to be operationalised, and the interview techniques for detecting them standardised, as preliminaries to the rigorous definition of appropriate criteria for caseness. Related to this, and discussed in more detail in Chapter 2, is the selection of instruments for detecting cases. The techniques most widely used in epidemiological surveys are questionnaires, semi-structured interviews and unstructured psychiatric interviews. The elderly have particular difficulties in reading, understanding and responding appropriately to questionnaires and the results of interviews may be influenced considerably by the training and personality of the interviewer. The high prevalence of both acute and chronic physical illness among the elderly can make the distinction between physical and psychiatric symptoms difficult, even for the experienced interviewer. Most community studies, however, use data collected by lay interviewers, who may not have adequate training in distinguishing significant depressive symptoms from the physical problems and dissatisfactions often experienced by elderly people. Although some of the commonly used rating scales for depression may be sufficient to generate DSM III (American Psychiatric Association 1980) or DSMIIR (American Psychiatric Association 1987) diagnoses, they do not, for the most part, address the symptoms most characteristic of depression in old age. It is clearly necessary to ensure that measures used in the epidemiological study of depression in old age are both valid and reliable in the specific population being examined.

Many elderly subjects complain of hypochondriacal symptoms or sleep disturbance rather than depressed mood. The effect of this can be minimised by the inclusion of a separate 'somatic symptoms' rating scale, as incorporated in the diagnostic schedule of Copeland et al. (1986). The clinical distinction, within a brief screening questionnaire or interview, between depression and dementia may be a further problem, resulting in considerable risk of demented subjects contaminating a survey-identified 'elderly depressed' sample.

Response bias is a further problem in epidemiological surveys of elderly people in whom a relatively high refusal rate is common. Rockwood et al (1989) noted that non-responders to a health status survey used significantly more health service resources and in particular had more hospital admissions. More specifically, Livingston et al. (1990), in a survey in which particular care was taken to recruit subjects initially reluctant to participate, found that depression, unlike dementia, was less frequently found in subjects recruited with difficulty.

Most epidemiological studies have attempted to identify representative samples within the community; others have examined samples within residential care settings or, following the recommendation of Freedman et al. (1982), attending their family physician. Community and special setting samples are discussed separately below. Studies of depression in the physically ill elderly are reviewed in Chapter 5.

COMMUNITY-BASED STUDIES

Kay and Bergmann (1980) have reviewed several early studies that relied mainly on open-ended clinical interviews and on short symptom questionnaires. The main conclusions to emerge from these studies are that, with increasing age, depression becomes the most prevalent neurosis, although psychotic affective illness in old age is relatively rare. Bergmann (1971), in a study of neurosis in old age, showed that whilst anxiety was the most common disorder in the 'chronic' neurotic group, depression was far commoner among 'late onset' neurotics. These studies confirm the findings of the classic paper by Kay et al. (1964) in which mild degrees of 'affective disorders and neuroses' were found in 16.2% and moderate to severe such disorders in 10%. It proved impossible to distinguish accurately between endogenous and reactive depressions but the prevalence of 'endogenous affective disorder' was estimated at 1.3% to 3%, depending on whether past psychiatric history was taken into account. The findings of a study of volunteers by Gianturco and Busse (1978) are similar. They studied 264 subjects aged 60 and over who were willing to complete interviews and clinical examinations lasting two days as part of a longitudinal study of aging. Although they attempted to make their sample demographically representative of the local population in Durham, North Carolina, the sample may well have been biased by the self-selection of volunteers for such detailed interviews. No information was given as to criteria for assessing depression, but 21% of subjects were recorded as being depressed.

More recent studies can usefully be divided into those using self-completed rating scales; those based on brief interviewer-completed scales; and those in which a detailed interview enables formal diagnoses based on standardised criteria to be made.

STUDIES USING SELF-COMPLETED RATING SCALES

Raymond et al. (1980), using the Wakefield Scale (Snaith et al. 1971), which does not include any of the depressive features particularly associated with old age depression, found a prevalence of significant depressive symptomatology in 34.5% of a randomly selected community sample, with a refusal rate of only 12.5%.

Kivela et al. (1986) reported a follow-up study of a sample of Finnish men previously examined in middle age. It is unclear how representative the initial sample was, but 93% of survivors were available for follow-up and, using the Zung Self-rating Depression Scale (SDS; Zung 196) with a cut-off point of 60 points or over, a prevalence of depression of 7% was found. A stratified random sample of elderly Swiss subjects by Lalive D'Epinay (1985) used the Wang Depression Scale (Wang et al. 1975). No information is given as to the criteria used for defining depressed subjects, but 28% overall scored 'high' on the scale.

Blazer and Williams (1980) administered detailed standardised questionnaires to 997 (85% of the total sample approached) subjects in Durham, North Carolina. They extracted 7 items from the questionnaire that enabled an assessment of dysphoric mood, and identified a further 11 items that allowed a DSM III diagnosis of major depressive illness to be made or excluded: 14.7% of subjects had dysphoric mood but only 3.7% fulfilled criteria for major depressive episode. The authors further analysed the 11% of their sample who, while showing significantly dysphoric mood, did not fulfil DSM III criteria for major depressive episode. Of these 110 subjects, 45 exhibited a pure dysphoria syndrome, the remainder having dysphoric mood in the setting of significant physical illness.

A number of American studies hue used the Centre for Epidemiological Studies Depression Scale (CES-D; Radloff 1977) to screen for depression in very large elderly community samples. Murrell et al. (1983) studied a total sample of 2517 subjects aged 55 and over. Laudably, they presented their data stratified in age bands, reporting an overall prevalence of depression of 17.5% in their subsample aged 65 and over. Their overall response rate was 80%. More recently, Blazer et al.

(1991) examined 3998 (80% of an original randomly selected age and sex strati-fied sample) of community-dwelling subjects aged 65 and over, and found 9% overall to score over the depression cut-off (CES-D total > 16). The proportion in the depressed range was higher for women and for the over 85s. Kennedy et al. (1989) reported a somewhat higher overall prevalence of high CES-D scores in a similarly stratified sample, with 17% (11% of men and 20% of women) scoring within the depressed range.

Fuhrer et al. (1992) examined a large (n = 2792) sample of subjects aged 65 and over in south-west France using the CES-D with a modified cut-off of 17 (men) and 23 (women) for significant depressive symptomatology. They reported an overall prevalence of depression of 15.9%.

STUDIES USING BRIEF INTERVIEWER-COMPLETED SCALES

Griffith et al. (1987) sought volunteers among a sample of 1500 mobile elderly subjects identified from general practice registers. They used a structured inter-view to elicit the symptoms listed in the Hamilton Depression Rating Scale (HDRS; Hamilton 1960) and, with a cut-off of 13 points or over to identify depression, reported an overall prevalence of 8%. This result is difficult to inter-pret since, as the authors themselves point out, the scale they used was intended specifically for measuring severity of depression in a sample already diagnosed clinically as suffering from a depressive illness.

Morgan et al. (1987) interviewed a stratified sample of elderly subjects in Nottingham using a structured interview incorporating the Symptoms of Anxiety and Depression Scale (SAD: Bedford et al. 1976). They found a prevalence of depression of 10 % using the criteria of a total SAD score greater than 6 and a depression subscale score of 4 or more. These criteria for depression agreed poorly with clinical ratings in a small subsample. A more conservative cut-off (total SAD >7 and depressive subscale >6) maximised agreement with clinical judgment, and gave a prevalence for depression of 4.9%.

STUDIES USING DIAGNOSTIC INTERVIEWS (see Table 3.1)

Two major studies have used the Present State Examination (PSE; Wing et al. 1974), a detailed interview schedule and associated CATEGO computerised diag-nostic algorithm. Ben-Arie et al. (1987) examined a random community sample of 139 coloured persons aged 65 and over in Capetown, South Africa, having excluded demented subjects (using the Mini-Mental State Examination, MMSE, of Folstein et al. 1975) and those with diagnoses other than depression. Twenty-three (16.5%) had sufficient depressive symptomatology to enable a tentative CATEGO diagnosis of depression to be made. Full psychiatric interviewing of these subjects confirmed the diagnosis of depression in 19, giving a prevalence rate of clinically confirmed depression of 13.7%. Six subjects had 'threshold' levels of depression and 13 definite depression. In close agreement with this, Carpiniello

Table 3.1 Interview-based community studies

Study	Diagnostic criteria	n	Age	'Major' depression (%)	'Minor' depression (%)
Kat et al. (1985)	AGECAT	274	70 +	14.2	
Copeland et al. (1987b) (London)	AGECAT	396	65 +	3.3	16.2
Copeland et al. (1987b) (New York)	AGECAT	445	65 +	1.8	14.4
Copeland et al. (1987a)	AGECAT	1070	65 +	2.9	8.3
Ben-Arie et al. (1987)	CATEGO	139	65 +	9.4	4.3
Kivela et al. (1988)	DSM III	1529	60 +	3.7	23.2
Bland et al. (1988)	DSM III	358	65 +	3.2	3.7
Lindesay et al. (1989)	SHORT-CARE	890	65 +	4.3	9.2
Carpiniello et al. (1989)	CATEGO	317	65 +	11.0	
Magnusson (1989)	AGECAT	876	87	7.8	
Livingston et al. (1990)	SHORT-CARE	705	65 +	15.9	
Madianos et al. (1992)	DSM III	251	65 +	2.2	7.5
Heeren et al. (1992)	DSM III	1259	85 +	7.1	
Skoog (1993)	DSM IIIR	494	85 +	13.6	5.9

The categories 'major' and 'minor' depression summarise the division into subtypes within the various diagnostic systems. For DSM III and DSM IIIR 'major' corresponds to major depressive syndrome and bipolar disorder and 'minor' to all other categories of affective disorder. For AGECAT, 'major' corresponds to depressive psychosis and 'minor' to depressive neurosis.

et al. (1989), who used a short community version of the PSE in a random sample of 317 subjects aged 65 or over (302 of whom agreed to participate) in Sardinia, reported that 14% were clinically depressed.

Myers et al. (1984) reported the findings of the Epidemiologic-Catchment-Area (ECA) study, which used a structured clinical interview to elicit the prevalence of a range of DSM III diagnoses in over 9000 adults. In the subsample aged 65 and over, the overall prevalence of affective disorder of any kind (using DSM III criteria) was 2.7%, and that of major depressive episode was 1%. A further 1.5% of their sample fulfilled DSM III criteria for dysthymia ('chronic mild depression'). Their interview schedules did not, however, include information on current duration of symptoms and their dysthymia figures refer to dysthymia at any time in the individuals' lives rather than in the immediate past two years.

A very large Finnish study by Kivela et al. (1988) surveyed the entire population (n = 1529) aged 65 and over of a semi-idustrialised municipality, using the SDS as a screening instrument and administering a clinical interview that elicited DSM IIIR diagnoses to high scorers and a random sample of low scorers. Major depression was present in 2.6% of men and 4.5% of women, with a further 2% of both genders fulfilling criteria for atypical depression. Dysthymia was however present in as many as 17% of men and 23% of women.

Bland et al. (1988) found that only 4.5% of elderly subjects in Edmonton, Canada, fulfilled DSM III criteria for affective disorder. In keeping with several of the other studies summarised above, they found that only about one-third of them (1.2% of the total sample) had major depression, most of the remainder fulfilling criteria for dysthymia. Madianos et al. (1992) reported a somewhat higher prevalence of DSM III affective disorder (9.5%) among elderly community-dwelling subjects in Athens. Here too, only very few (1.5%) had major depression.

Two very recent studies have examined very old (85 +) subjects. Heeren et al. (1992) used DSM III criteria and found an overall prevalence (major depression and dysthymia combined) of 3.7%. In contrast, Skoog (1993), who used DSM IIIR criteria, found the prevalence of affective disorder as a whole to be 19.8%. Surprisingly, the majority of cases fulfilled criteria for major depression rather than dysthymia.

The above studies did not use interview schedules specifically designed for elderly subjects. As discussed in Chapter 2, a number of such interview schedules, notably the CARE and its shorter versions and the GMS, are, however, now available for epidemiological studies of depression in old age.

Two recent British studies have used the depression schedule of the SHORT-CARE and reported broadly compatible results. Livingston et al. (1990) studied an electoral-ward-based sample in north London and took particular care to maximise the accuracy of the sample identified and the response rate. 17.3% were found to have probable 'pervasive depression' by which the authors meant depression of a severity in which specific therapeutic intervention would have been appropriate. A small number of depressed subjects also had a primary diagnosis of dementia; their exclusion gave a corrected pure depression prevalence of 15.9%. The female/male ratio was about 1.5:1 except in subjects aged 80 and over, in whom no sex difference was apparent. Only 13% of those found to be depressed (and 3% of those not depressed) were being treated with anti-depressants, although depression was associated with more frequent contact with the general practitioner.

In a south London sample of 890 subjects with a very high (86%) response rate, Lindesay et al. (1989) took particular care to distinguish between diagnoses of depression and anxiety. Prevalence rates for depression were very similar in the young-old and old-old, with overall rates of 8.4% in men and 11.3% in women. Interestingly, severe depression was equally common in men and women, the overall excess in women being accounted for entirely by milder cases.

Several studies have used the GMS. Kay et al. (1985) examined a random sample of subjects aged 70 and over in Hobart, Tasmania, and were able to generate both AGECAT and DSM III diagnoses. They reported moderate to severe depression on the AGECAT system in 14.2% of subjects and DSM III major depression in 10.2%. A further 19% of their subjects had significantly dysphoric mood but did not fulfil DSM III criteria for major depression. Kay et al. (1985) commented that this large subsample 'must include dysthymia disorder proper', but unfortunately did not present data on how many subjects fulfilled DSM III criteria for dysthymia. Though noting that their reported prevalence rate for DSM III major depression was higher than that of most comparable studies, the authors provided little explanation for this. They stressed that the symptoms of poor sleep, reduced energy, etc., that are crucial to DSM III diagnoses were reported very frequently in their sample, whereas thoughts of guilt and suicide were relatively rare.

Copeland et al. (1987b) reported AGECAT prevalence of 16.2% in a New York sample of 445 subjects aged 65 and over, and 19.5% in a London sample of 396 subjects. Prevalence for depressive psychosis were much lower, at 1.85% and 3.3% respectively. DSM III diagnoses were also available for the London sample, 4.6% having major affective disorder, 6.3% dysthymia and an additional 1.8% suffering from bereavement reactions. A further study by Copeland et al. (1987a) of 1070 subjects in Liverpool reported a prevalence of depressive illness of 11.3%, 2.9% with psychotic features. More recently, Magnusson (1989) studied a sample of very elderly (87-year-old) subjects in Iceland using the GMS, and reported an overall prevalence of 7.8%.

It is clear that there is considerable discrepancy between the relatively low prevalence in most studies of DSM III or DSM IIIR major depressive illness on the one hand, and the high rates of depressive symptomatology and of depressive diagnoses according to criteria specific for the elderly on the other. One factor relevant to this discrepancy is the problem of depression-like clinical features, such as fatigue, changes in sleep pattern and increasing physical ill health, associated with normal aging. Even allowing for this, however, the evidence is overwhelming that a considerable proportion of elderly subjects have genuine and disabling depressive symptoms that do not fit into the rubric of major depression according to the criteria of DSM III or DSM IIIR. The evidence from studies that have examined a broader range of DSM diagnoses suggests that many of these subjects fulfil the criteria for dysthymia.

STUDIES IN RESIDENTIAL SETTINGS

A number of studies have estimated the prevalence of depression in elderly people in institutional settings. The early study of Kay et al. (1964) reported an extremely low prevalence of affective illness and neurosis in the institutionalised elderly. Phillips and Henderson (1991) have reviewed a total of 17 epidemiological surveys of depression in elderly nursing home residents and found reported prevalence ranging between 5% and 85%. This variability must to some extent be a reflection of differing diagnostic criteria. A consistent trend may however be seen for more recent studies to report considerably higher levels of depression in residential settings than in the community. This most likely represents differences in admission practices to such residential care over the past 20 years. Though originally set up to provide hotel-type care for elderly people with mild degrees of physical frailty, residential homes have gradually come to be used almost exclusively by people with severe mental and/or physical disabilities. A number of relatively recent and large-scale studies are discussed in more detail below.

In a study of 300 white residents of old age homes in South Africa, Gillis and Zabow (1982) found that 10% not only scored high on a measure of poor life satisfaction, but had HDRS scores of greater than 15, indicating at least moderate depression. A further 16.6% had high scores on poor life satisfaction only, and were categorised as 'dysphoric'.

Several studies have used the depression scale from the SHORT-CARE interview (Gurland et al. 1984) to obtain more standardised depression ratings. Macdonald and Dunn (1982) studied 633 old people's home residents and elderly inpatients and day patients at psychiatric hospitals. Depression ratings could be performed on 397, and the prevalence of depression was 19.1%.

In Milan, Spagnoli et al. (1986) reported a higher prevalence of depression. They examined 368 elderly subjects randomly selected from the residents of the city's residential homes. The depression scale was given to the 75% of the sample with adequate cognitive functioning. Of these, 34% scored within the depressed range, giving a corrected prevalence for depression of 30%.

Harrison et al. (1990) surveyed 1303 of the 1471 residents in receipt of local-authority-provided home care and in a range of residential settings (including private as well as local authority residential homes and warden-assisted accommodation) using the depression subscale of the SHORT-CARE. Depression was commonest among those living in their own homes but receiving care (44%) and those in warden-assisted accommodation (43%). Depression was, however, also present in as many as 35% of those in private residential care and 28% of those in local authority provided residential care. The validity of the diagnoses of depression was attested to by the fact that a past history of depression was recorded twice as often in depression-positive subjects than in subjects without current evidence of depression.

Mann et al. (1984) surveyed all the residents of old people's homes in Camden, North London, using the depression and organic brain syndrome subscales of the SHORT-CARE. They were able to interview 82% of the total population of 535 subjects. One-third of these were severely demented, and of the 289 subjects in whom depression ratings were obtainable, 38% showed significant depressive symptomatology. Ames (1990) has recently replicated these findings in Camden, with the further step of full clinical interview in subjects identified on screening as positive for depression. A total of 15.6% fulfilled criteria for DSM III depressive disorder (9.2% for major depressive disorder).

Two other studies were also able to obtain standardised diagnostic information. Parmelee et al. (1989) interviewed 708 from a total of 1133 residents of a large facility for Jewish aged which incorporated a sheltered housing unit and a nursing home. The majority of those not seen were excluded because of cognitive or hearing impairment. Even within the successfully interviewed sample, significant cognitive deficits were present in 39%, reflecting the high level of dependency of such a population. 12% of subjects fulfilled DSM III criteria for major depression, with a further 30% having significant depressive symptomatology. Little difference in prevalence of depression was found between those with and without cognitive deficits.

Phillips and Henderson (1991) carried out a survey of 323 residents (a random 1-in-2 sample) of 24 nursing homes, using a clinical interview schedule designed to elicit diagnoses of depression both on DSM IIIR and on the then current draft of ICD10 (World Health Organisation 1992). Only 51% of subjects had sufficiently well-preserved cognitive functioning to score 18 or more on the MMSE and thereby to allow the depression interview to be performed. Of these 9.7% fulfilled DSM IIIR criteria for major depression and a further 3.6% for dysthymia. A somewhat higher proportion (21%) fulfilled ICD10 criteria, split roughly equally between severe, moderate and mild.

STUDIES IN PRIMARY CARE

Macdonald (1986) examined a random sample of elderly general practice attenders, using the SHORT-CARE interview. Only 10% of the total sample of 235 subjects refused to be interviewed, and a prevalence of depression of 30.6% was reported. The same instrument was used by Iliffe et al. (1991) in a random sample of 236 patients aged 75 and over identified through general practitioner lists and interviewed at home. 21.2% of the sample (13.4% of men and 26.9% of women) had significant depression, which in almost all cases was mild to moderate in severity. Only three patients from the whole sample had 'depression' recorded in their case notes, and six were being treated with antidepressants. Oxman et al. (1990) used the CES-D as well as depression-related items from the Hopkins symptom checklist (Derogatis et al. 1973) to elicit Research Diagnostic Criteria (RDC; Spitzer and Endicott 1978) diagnoses in consecutive patients attending their primary care physician. Of the 92 subjects aged 60 and over, 19 (21%) fulfilled criteria for major depressive disorder. Evans and Katona (1993) screened a series of elderly GP attenders using the GDS and recorded a prevalence of 36% (30% in men and 40% in women). A sub sample in whom GDS diagnoses were validated with the GMS interview yielded a corrected prevalence of 37%, almost all the interview-positive subjects having an AGECAT diagnosis of depressive neurosis. A considerably lower rate for depression as detected with the GDS (18%) was, however, found by Jack et al. (1988) in British primary care attenders aged 75 and over.

CONCLUSIONS

Two main conclusions emerge from the epidemiological studies reviewed in this hapter. The first is that significant depressive symptomatology (as measured by clinical interview schedules designed specifically for use with the elderly or by combining all categories of affective disorder within standard diagnostic systems) is at least as common as in young or middle-aged subjects and much more prevalent than suggested by the statistics for DSM III or DSM IIIR major depression. Particularly in the light of the findings of Kivela et al. (1989), discussed in Chapter 1, that the major depression/dysthymia split does not reflect severity in older subjects, it is regrettable that the challenge of incorporating the different clinical characteristics of depression in old age has not been taken up either in ICD10 or, in all probability, in the forthcoming DSM IV.

Second, it seems clear that, although reported rates of depression vary quite widely between the studies cited above, both elderly subjects in residential settings and those attending their general practitioners show rates of significant depressive symptomatology somewhat higher than those reported from community samples. This probably reflects the greater prevalence of both social and biological risk factors for depression (see Chapter 4) both in institutionalised elderly subjects and in those needing to make frequent visits to their primary care physician. In clinical practice, however, rates of both detection and active treatment of such depression are low in these 'high-risk' groups. This strongly suggests that elderly people in residential care, and more particularly those attending their GP, are subjects in whom active screening for depression and subsequent treatment where appropriate could be most rewarding.

REFERENCES

American Psychiatric Association (1980) *Diagnostic and Statistical Manual of Mental Disorders* (3rd edn). Washington, American Psychiatric Association.

American Psychiatric Association (1987) *Diagnostic and Statistical Manual of Mental Disorders* (3rd edn, revised). Washington, American Psychiatric Association.

Ames D (1990) Depression among elderly residents of local-authority residents homes: its nature and the efficacy of intervention. *British Journal of Psychiatry* 156, 667–76.

Bedford A, Foulds GA and Sheffield BF (1976) A new personal disturbance scale. *British Journal of Social and Clinical Psychology* 15, 387–94.

Ben-Arie O, Swarte L and Dickman BJ (1987) Depression in the elderly living in the community: its presentation and features. *British Journal of Psychiatry* 150, 169–74.

Bergmann K (1971) The neuroses of old age. In Kay DWK and Walk A (eds) *Recent Developments in Psychogeriatrics: A Symposium. British Journal of Psychiatry*, Special Publication No. 6.

Bland RC, Newman SC and Orn H (1988) Prevalence of psychiatric disorders in the elderly in Edmonton. *Acta Psychiatrica Scandinavica* 77 (Suppl. 338), 57–63.

Blazer D, Birchett B, Service C and George LC (1991) The association of age and depression among the elderly: an epidemiologic exploration. *Journal of Gerontology* 46, M210–15.

Blazer D and Williams CD (1980) Epidemiology of dysphoria and depression in an elderly population. *American Journal of Psychiatry* 137, 439–44.

Carpiniello B, Carta MG and Rudas N (1989) Depression among elderly people: a psychosocial study of urban and rural populations. *Acta Psychiatrica Scandinavica* 80, 445–50.

Copeland JRM (1981) What is a case, a case for what? In King JR, Bebbington P and Robins LN (eds) *What is a Case? The Problems of Definition in Psychiatric Community Surveys.* London, Grant McIntyre.

Copeland JRM, Dewey ME and Griffiths-Jones HM (1986) A computerized psychiatric diagnostic system and case nomenclature for elderly subjects: GMS and AGECAT. *Psychological Medicine* 16, 89–99.

Copeland JRM, Dewey ME, Wood N et al. (1987a) Range of mental illness among the elderly in the community: prevalence in Liverpool using the GMS-AGECAT package. *British Journal of Psychiatry* 150, 815–23.

Copeland JRM, Gurland BJ, Dewey ME et al. (1987b) Is there more dementia, depression and neurosis in New York? A comparative community study of the elderly in New York and London using the community diagnosis AGECAT. *British Journal of Psychiatry* 151, 466–73.

Derogatis LR, Lipman RS, Rickels K et al. (1973). The Hopkins Symptom Checklist (HSCL): a measure of primary symptom dimensions. In Pulot P (ed) *Psychological Measurement: Problems in Psychopharmacotheropy.* Basel, Karger.

Evans S and Katona CLE (1993) Prevalence of depressive symptoms in elderly primary care attenders. *Dementia*, in press.

Folstein MF, Folstein SE and McHugh PR (1975) 'Mini-Mental State': a practical method for grading the cognitive state of patients for the clinican. *Journal of Psychiatric Research* 12, 189–98.

Freedman N, Bucci W and Elkowitz E (1982) Depression in a family practice elderly population. *Journal of the American Geriatrics Society* 30, 372–7.

Fuhrer R, Antonucci TC, Gagnon M et al. (1992) Depressive symptomatology and cognitive functioning: an epidemiological survey in an elderly community sample in France. *Psychological Medicine* 22, 159–72.

Gianturco DT and Busse EW (1978) Psychiatric problems encountered during a long-term study of normal aging volunteers. In Issacs AD and Post F (eds) *Studies in Geriatric Psychiatry.* New York, John Wiley.

Gillis, LS and Zabow A (1982) Dysphoria in the elderly. *South African Medical Journal* 62, 410–13.

Griffiths RA, Good WR, Watson NP et al. (1987) Depression, dementia and disablity in the elderly. *British Journal of Psychiatry* 150, 482–93.

Gurland BJ, Golden RR, Teresi JA and Challop J (1984) The SHORT-CARE: an efficient instrument for the assessment of depession, dementia and disability. *Journal of Gerontology* 39, 166–9.

Hamilton M (1960) A rating scale for depression. *Journal of Neurology, Neurosurgery and Psychiatry* 23, 56–62.

Harrison R, Savla N and Kafetz K (1990) Dementia, depression and physical disability in a London borough: a survey of elderly people in and out of residential care and implications for future developments. *Age and Ageing*, 19, 97–103.

Heeren TJ, van Hemert AM, Lagaay AM and Rooymans HGM (1992) The general population prevalence of non-organic psychiatric disorders in subjects aged 85 years and over. *Psychological Medicine* 22, 733–8.

Iliffe S, Haines A, Gallivan S et al. (1991) Assessment of elderly people in general practice 1. Social circumstances and mental state. *British Journal of General Practice* 41, 9–12.

Jack MA, Stobo SA, Scott LA et al. (1988) Prevalence of depression in general practice patients over 75 years of age. *Journal of the Royal College of General Practitioners* 38, 20–1.

Jacoby RJ and Levy R (1980) Computed tomography in the elderly: 3. Affective disorder. *British Journal of Psychiatry* 136, 270–5.

Kay DWK, Beamish P and Roth M (1964) Old age mental disorders in Newcastle upon Tyne. Part I: A study of prevalence. *British Journal of Psychiatry* 110, 146–58.

Kay DWK and Bergmann K (1980) Epidemiology of mental disorders among the aged in the community. In Birren JE and Slone RB (eds) Handbook of Mental Health and Ageing. Englewood Cliffs, NJ, Prentice-Hall.

Kay DWK, Henderson AS, Scott R et al. (1985) Dementia and depression among the elderly living in the Hobart community: the effect of diagnostic criteria on the prevalence rates. Psychological Medicine 15, 771–8.

Kennedy GJ, Kelman HR, Thomas C et al. (1989) Hierarchy of characteristics associated with depressive symptoms in an urban elderly sample. American Journal of Psychiatry 146, 220–7.

Kivela S-L, Nissinen A, Tuomilehto J et al. (1986) Prevalence of depressive and other symptoms in elderly Finnish men. Acta Psychiatrica Scandinavica 73, 93–100.

Kivela S-L, Pahkala K and Laippala P (1988) Prevalence of depression in an elderly population in Finland. Acta Psychiatrica Scandinavica 78, 401–13.

Kivela S-L, Palskala K and Eronen P (1989) Depressive symptoms and signs that differentiate major and atypical depression from dysthymic disorder in elderly Finns. International Journal of Geriatric Psychiatry 4, 79–85.

Lalive D'Epinay CJ (1985) Depressed elderly women in Switzerland: an example of testing and generating theories. The Gerontologist 25, 597–604.

Lindesay J, Briggs K and Murphy E (1989) The Guy's/Age Concern Survey: prevalence rates of cognitive impairment, depression and anxiety in an urban elderly community. British Journal of Psychiatry 155, 317–29.

Livingston G, Hawkins A, Graham N et al. (1990) The Gospel Oak Study: prevalence rates of dementia, depression and activity limitation among elderly residents in inner London. Psychological Medicine 20, 137–46.

Macdonald AJD (1986) Do general practitioners 'miss' depression in elderly patients? British Medical Journal 292, 1365–7.

Macdonald AJD and Dunn J (1982) Death and the expressed wish to die in the elderly: an outcome study. Age ad Ageing, 11, 189–95.

Madianos MG, Gournas G and Stefanis CN (1992) Depressive symptoms and depression among elderly people in Athens. Acta Psychiatrica Scandinavica 86, 320–6.

Magnusson H (1989) Mental health of octogenarians in Iceland. An epidemiological study. Acta Psychiatrica Scandinavica 79, Suppl. 349.

Mann AH, Graham N and Ashby D (1984) Psychiatric illness in residential homes for the elderly: a survey in one London borough. Age and Ageing 13, 257–65.

Morgan K, Dallosso HM, Arie T et al. (1987) Mental health and psychological well-being among the old and the very old living at home. British Journal of Psychiatry 150, 801–7.

Murrell SA, Himmelfarb SA and Wright K (1983) Prevalence of depression and its correlates in older adults. American Journal of Epidemiology 117, 173–85.

Myers JK, Weissman MM, Tischler GL et al. (1984) Six-month prevalence of psychiatric disorders in three communities. Archives of General Psychiatry 41, 959–67.

Oxman TE, Barrett-JE, Barrett J and Gerber P (1990) Symptomatology of late-life minor depression among primary care patients. Psychosomatics 31, 174–80.

Parmelee PA, Katz IR and Lawton MP (1989) Depression among institutionalised aged: assessent and prevalence estimation. Journal of Gerontology, M22–9.

Phillips CJ and Henderson AS (1991) The prevalence of depression among Australian nursing home residents: results using draft ICD-10 and DSM-III-R criteria. Psychological Medicine 21, 739–48.

Post F and Shulman K (1985) New views on old age affective disorders. In Arie T (ed.) Recent Developments in Psychogeriatrics, no. 1. Churchill Livingstone, London.

Raymond EF, Michals TJ and Steer RA 1980) Prevalence and correlates of depression in elderly persons. Psychological Reports 47, 1055–61.

Radloff LS (1977) The CES-D scale: a self-rating depression scale for research in the general population. *Applied Psychological Measurement* 1, 385–401.

Rockwood K, Stolee P, Robertson D and Shillington ER (1989) Response bias in a health status survey of elderly people. *Age and Ageing* 18, 177–82.

Skoog I (1993) The prevalence of psychotic, depressive and anxiety syndromes in demented and non-demented 85-year-olds. *International Journal of Geriatric Psychiatry* 8, 247–253.

Snaith RP, Ahmed SN, Mehta S and Hamilton M (1971) Assessment of the severity of primary depressive illness: the Wakefield self-assessment depression inventory. *Psychological Medicine* 1, 143–9.

Spagnoli A, Foresti G, Macdonald A et al. (1986) Dementia and depression in Italian geriatric institutions. *International Journal of Geriatric Psychiatry* 1, 15–23.

Spitzer RL and Endicott J (1978) *Research Diagnostic Criteria for a Selected Group of Functional Disorders* (3rd edn) New York, New York State Psychiatric Institute.

Wang R, Trubs S and Alberno L (1975) A brief self-assessing depression scale. *Journal of Clinical Pharmacology* 15, 163–7.

Wing JK, Cooper JE and Sartorius N (1974) *The Measurement and Classification of Psychiatric Symptoms*. Cambridge, Cambridge University Press.

World Health Organisation (1992) *The ICD-10 Classification of Mental and Behavioural Disorders: Clinical Descriptions and Diagnostic Guidelines*. Geneva, World Health Organisation.

Zung WK (1965) A self-rating depression scale. *Archives of General Psychiatry* 12, 63–6.

4 The Aetiology of Depression in Old Age

An understanding of the possible aetiological factors underlying depression in old age is not only necessary to explain the relatively high overall prevalence of depressive symptomatology in old age, but should also be helpful in identifying those at particularly high risk and enable intervention strategies to be generated. The majority of studies to date have focused on broadly social or broadly biological factors although there have been some attempts to generate integrated aetiological hypotheses. In this chapter, the possible roles of demographic, social and biological factors in predisposing elderly subjects to become depressed, in precipitating or maintaining such depression, or in protecting from it, will be discussed in turn.

DEMOGRAPHIC FACTORS

AGE

As has already been discussed (see Chapter 3) apparent changes in the prevalence of depression in old age reflect changes in symptom pattern more than real changes in prevalence. The overall rate of depression found using diagnostic instruments appropriate to an elderly population reveal rates similar to those found in middle-aged and younger subjects. Aging does not, therefore, appear to be an important aetiological factor for depression throughout adult life, though it has been suggested that cohort effects may confound the relationship between age and depression. Burke et al. (1991) used data from the NIMH-ECA database to show that subjects born before 1917 were much less likely to have had depressive episodes before the age of 30 than cohorts with later dates of birth. Warshaw et al. (1991) have extended this work by examining onset rates in birth cohorts of first degree relatives of probands with affective disorders from the NIMH collaborative study of the psychobiology of depression and have included a six-year follow-up study of the relatives. Striking increases in the rate of diagnosis of major depressive disorders in the mid-1960s were noted in all cohorts, with a further increase in the mid-1970s. This effect was seen most strongly in younger cohorts. The authors conclude that their results reflect an age-period rather than an age-cohort effect.

It remains possible, however, that within elderly subjects age may nonetheless be an important predisposing factor for depression. Blazer et al. (1991), in a very large sample (3998) of community-dwelling subjects aged 65 and over, found that whereas only 8.1% of those aged 65–74 scored above the CES-D repression threshold, 10.3% of those aged 75–84 had scores above the cut-off, as did 12.3% of those 85 and over. In a subsequent multiple regression analysis, however, the association between age and depressive symptoms was reversed when major confounding variables (sex, income, physical disability, cognitive impairment and social support) were simultaneously controlled. In a community study in Finland, examining all persons born in 1923 or earlier, Pahkala et al. (1991) found the mean age for those identified as suffering from major depression was nearly three years greater than that of non-depressed persons ($p < 0.05$). Almost identical results from the United States were reported by Kennedy et al. (1990). Unlike Blazer et al. (1991), however, neither Pahkala et al. (1991) nor Kennedy et al. (1990) entered age as a variable in their subsequent multivariate analysis.

No consistent age-related difference in rate of significant depressive symptomatology was found by Lewinsohn et al. (1991) in three separate samples of community residents aged 50 and over. Similarly, Dean et al. (1990) found no linear or non-linear age effects of depressive symptomatology in a sample of 997 married and widowed community subjects aged 50 and over.

It thus appears that, at least within the elderly, age does not emerge consistently as an independent risk factor for depression.

GENDER

Most epidemiological studies (see Chapter 3) have reported a considerably greater prevalence of depressive symptomatology in elderly females than in elderly male subjects, thus suggesting that female gender predisposes towards depression in old age. The aetiological influence of gender on depression in old age does not, however, appear to be purely a direct one. Several studies have suggested that gender is an important intermediary variable in determining the extent to which vulnerability to social risk factors for depression is manifest. Kennedy et al. (1989) found a highly significant ($p < 0.0002$) association between depression and age in women but no such relationship in men. Subsequent stepwise regression analysis showed the effects of both age and gender to be very small once health and disability variables had been allowed for.

In a complex study attempting specifically to tease out the influence of both age and gender on social risk factors for depression, Lewinsohn et al. (1991) found that correlations between social variables and depression differed significantly between men and women in 12 of the 115 variables examined. Depression in women was associated with feelings of dissatisfaction with important life roles, with experiencing physical disease, and with marital conflict, to a much greater extent than was the case in men.

The well-established (see below) relationship between physical ill health and depression was found by Husaini et al. (1991) to be equally evident in males and females in a sample of 600 black elderly community residents. In contrast, Cadoret and Widmer (1988) examined a group of elderly patients with recent-onset life-threatening or severely debilitating illness and an age- and sex-matched control group. Depressive symptoms increased significantly in the group of ill male patients but not in the ill female patients. The increase in depression in the ill male group remained evident when controlling for other depression-linked variables such as nursing home placement, prior history of depression and recent stressful life events.

The influence of smoking and drinking on depression may also be gender dependent. Kivela and Pahkala (1991) found that women were more likely to be depressed if they did not smoke and did not drink, whereas in men they found no relationship between drinking and depression. Male smokers were, however, more likely to be depressed than male non-smokers. A report from the Liverpool Longitudinal Community Study of Depression in Old Age (Saunders et al. 1991), restricted to males, found that those with a history of heavy drinking for five years or more at some time in their lives had a risk of depression more than five times greater than those without such a history of heavy drinking.

FAMILY HISTORY

There is consistent evidence that a positive family history is an important predisposing factor for depression in old age. This is particularly so for subjects with bipolar affective disorder (Shulman 1992). As discussed in Chapter 1, however, the genetic contribution appears least important in those with unipolar depression who become depressed for the first time late in life (Alexopoulos 1989; Brodaty et al. 1991).

SOCIAL FACTORS

ILLNESS AND DISABILITY

An early study by Linn et al. (1980) found a small but statistically significant correlation ($r = 0.23$) between level of disability and degree of depressive symptomatology. In a similar but more detailed study, Murphy (1982) compared elderly depressed subjects (the majority of whom were psychiatric outpatient referrals) with age- and sex-matched community controls. Severe chronic health difficulties were present in 39% of controls compared with 26% of the normal elderly subjects ($p < 0.05$). The small subsample of elderly depressed subjects identified as community-onset cases rather than as psychiatric referrals showed a still more marked excess of chronic physical health difficulties.

In a much larger community sample of elderly residents, Kennedy et al. (1989) found that 30% of those with four or more medical conditions scored above the cut-off point for depression, compared with only 5% of those with no medical conditions. When depression scores were regressed against predictor variables, the contribution of health and disability to variance in depression remained highly significant ($p < 0.0002$). Similarly, in a recent primary-care based study, Evans and Katona (1993) found that depression (as measured by detailed psychiatric interview) was almost twice as common in primary care attenders with significant physical health problems than in those without. Similarly, Blazer et al. (1991) found that disability and chronic illness, analysed as separate variables, were both highly significantly associated ($p < 0.01$) with depression rating scores.

The studies described above have used cross-sectional data to examine the relationship between depression and illness and/or disability. This relationship can be examined more specifically through longitudinal follow-up studies of subjects initially identified as not depressed. Murrell et al. (1991) found that deterioration in health was significantly associated with the development of new symptoms of depression. They failed, however, to demonstrate any buffering effect of good physical health on life-event induced depression.

Several studies have examined the effects of disability as distinct from poor health. Smallegan (1989) found a significant relationship between level of disability (measured on a 13-question disability scale referring to the need for help with items such as bathing and safety) and level of depression ($p < 0.01$), despite the fact that a very low overall rate of depression was found in their sample of subjects volunteering for study. In a larger stratified community sample, Dean et al. (1990) found a similar relationship between disability in activities of daily living and depression, as did Phillips and Henderson (1991) in a nursing home cohort. In a recent report from the ECA project, Bruce and McNamara (1992) found both major depression and dysthymia to be more than twice as common in bed- or chair-bound elderly subjects than in the non-home-bound. The relationship with dysthymia, but not that with major depression, remained statistically significant after controlling for degree of physical ill health. Oxman et al. (1992) examined the influence of disability on depression prospectively through follow-up interview after a three-year interval on an institutionalised sample. Deterioration in functional ability between baseline and follow-up interviews was significantly ($p < 0.0001$) associated with increased depression. Physical illness thus emerges as a major factor both in precipitating and in maintaining depression in old age.

LIFE EVENTS

The potential for recent adverse life events to precipitate depression has been well documented. Murphy (1982) replicated the studies of Brown's group (Brown and Harris 1978) with elderly patients and matched controls, and found that 48% of the patients as compared with only 23% of controls had experienced at least one severe independent event (such as bereavement, life-threatening illness of someone close) in the year prior to onset of depression. Similar statistically significant differences were found in rates of chronic social difficulties (42% vs 19%). It should be noted that the single commonest and most clearly distinguishing life event in this study was personal physical illness, though the results remained statistically significant when this was excluded. In a recent study using very similar methodology, Emmerson et al. (1989) examined severe life events in the shorter three-month period prior to onset of illness or interview and found rates of 24% the depressed patients and 7% for the controls. The results for the full year (38 vs 19%) were very similar to those reported by Murphy (1982). In a much larger stratified community sample, Dean et al. (1990) found highly significant correlations between undesirable life event scores and depression scores, but did not report raw prevalence rates.

A number of studies have examined the influence of more specific life events on the onset of depression. Linn et al. (1980) found that deaths or accidents amongst relatives and friends, and arguments with family or close friends were most closely associated with depression. Smallegan (1989) confirmed the relationship between arguments and depression but also noted significant associations with moving house and change in marital status. In a larger community study in Canada, Stephenson-Cino et al. (1992) confirmed the overall relationship between life events and depression and found specific associations with bereavement and with recent illness of a friend or relative. Very similar associations between depression and serious illness and death among relatives and friends were reported by Pahkala et al. (1991).

The effect of intervening variables in buffering the extent to which life events trigger depression is of considerable interest. Murphy (1982) found the association between life events and depression to be maintained only in the subsample lacking an intimate relationship. In those with such a relationship, rates of depression did not differ significantly between those experiencing a severe life event or major difficulty and those without such a stress. A similar protective effect of intimacy against life-event-induced depression was reported by Evans and Katona (1993).

Bereavement

Not surprisingly, bereavement is the single life event most clearly implicated in precipitating depression in elderly subjects. Murphy (1982) found that 15% of her depressed sample compared with only 7% of controls had recently experienced the death of a spouse or child ($p < 0.05$). More recently and strikingly, Pahkala et al. (1991) found that only 2% of 330 non-depressed community subjects compared with 31% of 42 depressed subjects had recently experienced the death of a close friend or relative. Kennedy et al. (1989) found that the relative risk of depression was nearly twice as great in subjects who had experienced the death of a family member in the past six months than those spared such an experience. In a multiple regression analysis they found that the combined variable of family illness and bereavement remained a highly significant ($p = 0.0001$) associate of depression. They noted, however, that it explained only 2.9% of the variance, much less than the contribution of sleep disturbance or health and disability.

Prospective studies have also attempted to identify which bereaved subjects have higher risks of developing depression. In a two-year study of 189 widows and widowers, Zisook et al. (1987) found that subjects becoming depressed tended to be younger, to have been depressed in the past and to have experienced sudden and unanticipated bereavement rather than being bereaved after their spouse had had a long illness. In contrast, Hill et al. (1988) in a study of 95 widows, found no relationship between depression at one year and either expectedness of the bereavement or whether the subjects had mentally 'rehearsed' the death prior to it actually occurring. The discrepancy between these findings may be due to the relatively small number in the Hill et al. (1988) study. Dimond et al. (1987) examined the role of social support in a two-year prospective follow-up study of a group of elderly bereaved subjects (n = 192; mean age 67.6). By far the strongest predictor of depression at all time-points up to and including two years was severity of depression three weeks after bereavement. Quality of social network correlated modestly with depression at two months after bereavement but not later. Depression at two months also showed a small but statistically significant negative relationship with age and with length of marriage, but no such effect was found between either of these variables and later depression. Dimond et al. (1987) also failed to find any relationship between physical health and post-bereavement depression.

Perhaps the single clearest finding from these studies is that although depressive symptomatology is very common in the weeks immediately after bereavement, most subjects experience a gradual decrease in depressive symptoms without developing full-blown depressive illness. Persistent depression appears to be associated more with demographic and psychiatric variables (age, past history of depression) than with factors associated either with the marriage itself or with subsequent social support.

SOCIAL NETWORKS

Being married appears to protect against the development of depression in old age. Pahkala et al. (1991) found significantly higher rates of depression in subjects who were widowed or divorced. Similarly, Carpiniello et al. (1989) found that only 8% of their elderly subjects living in Sardinia were depressed compared with 17% of single subjects and 21% of those widowed (p < 0.01), and Stephenson-Cino et al. (1992) found only 5.6% of their married subjects scored above the CES-D depression cut-off compared with 11.4% of widows and 15.4% of separated or divorced subjects. In the latter study, the never-married group had a relatively low depression rate of 9%. Smallegan (1989) found depression to be associated both with lack of a spouse and with the experience of marital change.

Similar relationships have been demonstrated between a low level of social interaction and a higher risk of depression. Kennedy et al. (1990) found that living alone was associated with a more than two-fold increase in relative risk of depression; this finding was not confirmed in a sample of elderly primary care attenders (Evans and Katona, 1993). Pahkala et al. (1991) found significant relationships between depression and both living alone and decreased participation in social activities. A trend just failing to reach significance was found between depression and lack of intimate friends (19% vs 9%; $p < 0.06$). Husaini et al. (1991) reported a significant relationship in women but not in men between depression and reduced frequency of contact with relatives and friends. Prospective studies by Russell and Cutrona (1991) and by Oxman et al. (1992) both suggest that lack of social support predicts the subsequent development of depression; the latter study also found that worsening in level of social support between the baseline and follow-up interviews (three years later) also predicted the emergence of depression.

Quality of relationships may be more important in determining whether elderly subjects become depressed than 'harder' variables such as marital status, whether subjects live alone and number of social contacts per unit time. Murphy (1982) found that the absence of any confiding relationship was associated with depression rates at least double those found in subjects with at least some degree of intimate social contact, a finding replicated almost exactly in the community study of Kennedy et al. (1989).

Type of relationship and nature of social interaction are also relevant. Dean et al. (1990) found that availability of social support from spouses, friends and adult children (in that order) were important predictors of freedom from depression, but that support from other relatives was not associated with the presence or absence of depression. In an interesting small study of nursing home residents, Rotenberg and Hamel (1988) found that depression, though negatively correlated with a measure of quantity of more superficial social interactions, was *more* common in subjects with reciprocally intimate relationships. The authors hypothesised that whereas chatting protected against depression, more emotionally laden interactions might actually cause it.

Gender and life events may be important intermediate variables between intimacy and depression. Emerson et al. (1989) found the significant association between depression and the lack of a confiding relationship to be evident only in men. Fifty-seven per cent of depressed men and only 3% of male controls had no confidant, whereas in women the figures were 23% and 18%, respectively. Both Murphy (1982) and Evans and Katona (1993) found that the significant relationship between life events and depression in elderly subjects was only present in those without any confiding relationship.

FINANCIAL AND EDUCATIONAL STATUS

Several studies have noted a relationship between poverty and depression in old age. Dean et al. (1990) noted a significant direct effect of financial strain on depressive symptoms independent of the effect of life events and disability. Carpiniello et al. (1989) found a similar relationship between poverty and depression, which was, however, evident only in urban residents. Kennedy et al. (1989) found that subjects earning less than $5,000 a year had more than three times the risk of being depressed than those with incomes of more than $15,000 a year, but did not examine whether this association was independent of the many other psychosocial variables studied. In a follow-up study from the same sample, however, Kennedy et al. (1990) demonstrated that low income was significantly and independently associated with the emergence of new depression ($p < 0.02$). Low income also emerged as a significant and independent correlate with CES-D score in the community study by Blazer et al. (1991).

Education has received somewhat less attention as a possible correlate of depression in old age. Carpiniello et al. (1989) found an association between poor education and depression restricted to women and urban dwellers. Evans and Katona (1993) found a significant correlation between premorbid intelligence and questionnaire elicited depression scores but not with interview identified cases of depression.

PERSONALITY

Suprisingly few recent studies have examined personality variables in old age depression. Post and Shulman (1985) commented on the difficulty of defining personality in retrospect. In a long-term follow-up study, Ciompi (1969) reported that subjects with obsessional or hysterical premorbid personalities were more likely to have poor outcomes than those of impulsive personality.

The importance of personality variables in predisposing towards more minor depressive symptomatology (dysphoria) has been more extensively studied. Blazer and Williams (1980) found that alcohol abuse, use of analgesics and a perceived need for treatment for nerves were significantly commoner in elderly dysphorics than in the normal elderly, and concluded that dysphoria in old age is a reflection of 'decreased life satisfaction and periodic grief secondary to the physical, social, and economic difficulties encountered by aging individuals in the community'. Gillis and Zabow (1982) made detailed personality assessments on the basis of a close enquiry about past personality from relatives, friends and carers of their elderly subjects, and found that those with dysphoria exhibited 'life long manifestations of undue dependency, poor coping behaviour and inadequacy in inter-personal relationships'. They concluded that elderly dysphorics 'become increasingly like themselves'. Post and Shulman (1985), notwithstanding their misgivings about retrospective assessments of personality, emphasised the importance of 'innate and long standing personality factors' in the aetiology of dysphoria.

DEPRESSION IN ELDERLY CARERS

As many as 50% of the caregivers of people with Alzheimer's Disease meet standard criteria for depression (Gallagher et al. 1989). The emergence of such depression appears to depend on variables pertaining to both the carer and the demented patient. Schulz and Williamson (1991), in a two-year prospective study of caregivers of demented patients, found that female caregivers had significantly more severe depressive symptoms at baseline but showed little change in depression over the follow-up period. At baseline, 39% of female caregivers but only 16 of males scored above the CES-D cut-off for depression. Male carers, on the other hand, experienced steady increases in depression ratings with final mean scores much more similar to those of the female carers. Depression in caregivers was associated with behavioural problems in the patients they cared for, lack of perceived social support and poverty. There was also an association between a poor relationship with the demented patient prior to the onset of their dementia and the carer subsequently becoming depressed. The importance of family support for Alzheimer's disease caregivers was emphasised by Shields (1992), who found that 44% of the variance in caregivers' depressive symptoms was explained by angry and sad responses of extended family members to the caregiver.

Pruchno and Resch (1989) also found depression to be commoner in female than in male caregivers of subjects with Alzheimer's disease. In men, poor physical health was the sole predictor of depression, whereas in caregiving women, clear associations were found between depression and both poor health and lack of emotional investment in the caregiving task.

Gallagher et al. (1989), in a study of carers (mainly elderly spouses) of people with Alzheimer's disease, noted marked differences in rate of major depression between those who sought help to increase their coping skills (46%) and those identified in a longitudinal study of Alzheimer's disease (18%). Rates in both groups were much higher than might be expected in the population as a whole, but no differences in prevalence of depression were found related to gender or socioeconomic status of the carer, or to clinical characteristics of the person they were caring for. Drinka et al. (1987), in a broader-based study of caregivers of elderly male patients attending a geriatric referral clinic (73% of whom had dementia and 69% depression), found that caregiver depression was significantly correlated with patient depression but not with patient dementia or dependency. The overall prevalence of depression in this caregiver sample was very high at 83%. In view of the high prevalence and frequent chronicity of depression in old age, the implications of this study are important in highlighting the possible needs of the large population of caregivers of elderly depressed but not demented subjects.

BIOLOGICAL FACTORS

IMAGING

Structural

Interest in structural imaging in elderly depressed patients was considerably stimulated by the early finding by Jacoby and Levy (1980) that the CT scan appearances of elderly depressed patients were intermediate between those of subjects with dementia and of healthy elderly controls. Jacoby and Levy (1980) identified a small (n = 9) subgroup within their elderly depressed group with late age at first onset, relatively high age at time of scanning, endogenous symptom pattern and marked ventricular enlargement. No relationship was found, however, between degree of cognitive impairment and degree of ventricular enlargement. Subsequent follow-up (Jacoby et al. 1981) revealed that this subgroup also had a high mortality. Alexopoulos et al. (1992) confirmed the finding by Jacoby and Levy (1980) that depressed patients with first onset of illness at the age of 60 or older had greater ventricular size than those with earlier onset. The CT parameters in the latter group were similar to those of patients with Alzheimer's disease. Again, no relationship was found between severity of cognitive impairment within depression and CT parameters.

Two more recent studies have, however, established some links between cognitive and CT abnormalities within elderly depressed patients. Pearlson et al. (1989) examined elderly depressed patients with and without coexistent cognitive impairment. The latter group showed greater ventricular enlargement and decreased brain density. At two-year follow-up, however, only one of the 11 patients with depression-associated cognitive impairment had developed dementia. This suggests that though patients with depression-associated cognitive impairment may have underlying structural brain abnormalities, these are not necessarily precursors of irreversible degenerative brain disease. Somewhat different results were reported by Abas et al. (1990), who found no overall difference between elderly depressed and control subjects in ventricular–brain ratio, but did find significant correlations within the depressed group between cognitive test measures of slowing and degree of ventricular enlargement. They also demonstrated greater atrophy in patients with early rather than late age at first onset of depression and found particularly strong correlations between CT scan measures of atrophy and those psychological tests which showed persistent abnormality on recovery from depression.

Magnetic resonance imaging (MRI) has, as highlighted in the review by Baldwin (1993), recently provoked much interest as a more sensitive measure of structural change in elderly depressed patients. Such interest was stimulated by the finding (Coffey et al. 1988) that subcortical areas of white matter hyperintensity were frequently found in elderly depressed patients. A more recent study by the same group (Coffey et al. 1990) found, however, that similar hyperintensities were present in age-matched healthy controls. Both white matter hyperintensities and lesions of subcortical grey nuclei were more frequently found in the depressed group. In both groups, their presence was related to that of risk factors for vascular disease. Another study by the same group (Figiel et al. 1991) has reported that both caudate (60% vs 11%) and large deep white matter hyperintensities (also 60% vs 11%) were more frequent in subjects with late than in those with earlier first onset of depression. Rabins et al. (1991) found that elderly depressed subjects had a number of cortical as well as subcortical abnormalities. In particular, as well as subcortical white matter lesions, lesions in the basal ganglia were common and sulcal widening was evident particularly in the temporal cortex. The authors stress that theirs was the first study using MRI to demonstrate cortical as well as subcortical atrophy in elderly depressed patients. They failed, however, to replicate the relationship between white matter hyperintensities and vascular risk factors demonstrated by Coffey et al. (1990).

Functional

Functional imaging studies have involved measurement of regional cerebral blood flow (rCBF) by xenon (Xe) inhalation, single photon emission tomography (SPET) and positron emission tomography (PET). PET has also been used to measure glucose utilisation. Several Xe studies have reported abnormalities in cerebral blood flow in depression; none, however, has used a specifically elderly sample. Sackeim et al. (1990) reported overall reductions in rCBF in cognitively intact depressed subjects compared with matched controls, the reductions being most marked in frontal, anterior parietal and superior temporal regions. In contrast, Silfverskiold et al. (1989), who studied a relatively elderly (mean age 61) sample, did not find any overall difference in rCBF between depressed and control subjects. Within the depressed group, however, they found significant inverse correlations between rCBF and measures of depression, self-depreciation and cognitive dysfunction. They also found that rCBF did not increase with clinical improvement.

PET and SPET have been used relatively little in studies of elderly depressed patients. A SPET study by Beats and Levy (1992) showed reduced anterior frontal and anterior temporal blood flow as well as an increase in occipital cortex flow in elderly depressed patients. These findings are in keeping with a PET glucose metabolism study by Buschbaum et al. (1986), which showed reductions in frontal lobe glucose metabolism following an unpleasant electrical stimulus in younger bipolar patients. A very recent PET study (Bench et al. 1992) of middle-aged and elderly (mean age 56.8 years) depressed patients and matched controls, has found reductions in rCBF in left anterior cingulate and left dorso-lateral prefrontal cortex. Further abnormalities (significant decrease in rCBF in left medial frontal gyrus and increased rCBF in cerebellar vermis) were found in the subgroup of depressed patients with coexistent cognitive impairment. The authors suggest that the finding of both prefrontal and limbic (left anterior cingulate) anomalies might reflect the functional abnormality of an anatomical network in major depressive disorder.

NEUROENDOCRINE FUNCTION

Several aspects of neuroendocrine functioning have been studied in elderly depressed patients. The dexamethasone suppression test (DST), originally reported as being a highly sensitive and specific test for melancholia (Carroll et al.

1981), has received the most attention. Early reports suggested that age did not affect results either in control subjects (Carroll et al. 1981) or in depression (Carroll et al. 1981; Tourigny-Rivard et al. 1981). This was confirmed by Lewis et al. (1984) and by Molchan et al. (1990).

Both Georgotas et al. (1986) and Weiner et al. (1987) have, however, found higher rates of DST non-suppression in elderly than in younger volunteers. A number of studies in depressed patients also suggest that age may have an important mediating effect. Asnis et al. (1981) found a significant relationship between cortisol secretion and age in endogenous depression. Lewis et al. (1984) and Maes et al. (1991) both found a correlation between 8 a.m. post-dexamethasone cortisol and age in depressed patients; in the latter study, multiple regression analysis revealed age to be a highly significant mediator of cortisol secretion after dexamethasone. Relatively high rates of DST non-suppression in elderly depressed patients have been reported in several studies. Alexopoulos et al. (1984b) found that 80% of elderly subjects with endogenous depression compared with only 45% of younger subjects with the same diagnosis were non-suppressors. Similar findings were reported by Davis et al. (1984). Greden et al. (1986) also found high rates of DST suppression in older patients (71% in those aged over 70; 55% in the 40–70 age group; 50% in the under–40s). In this study, elderly non-suppressors were much less likely than their younger counterparts to show DST normalisation on clinical recovery as well as showing a poorer response to antidepressant drugs.

Greden et al. (1986) emphasised the importance, when comparing DST results in older and younger depressed subjects, of possible differences in severity or chronicity of depression. Molchan et al. (1990) found a significant positive relationship between severity of depression and post-dexamethasone cortisol in elderly depressed patients, though Davis et al. (1984) found no such relationship between DST result and either severity of depression or presence of psychotic features. Cognitive impairment may also be an important mediating variable. Siegel et al. (1989) found post-deamethasone cortisol levels to correlate with degree of cognitive impairment in elderly depressed patients, though no such correlation was found by Georgotas et al. (1986).

Other neuroendocrine probes have been studied relatively little in elderly depressed patients. The thyrotropin test (which is blunted in a proportion of patients with depression) is of considerable potential interest, however, since, unlike the DST, it appears to be free of marked age effects and to remain abnormal following clinical recovery (Loosen et al. 1987). Molchan et al. (1991b) found that elderly patients with major depression had lower TRH stimulated TSH levels than either controls or patients with Alzheimer's disease. No correlations were found between thyrotropin test results and severity of depression. The stability of thyrotropin test results with clinical recovery from depression has not been examined in a specifically elderly population. The same group (Molchan et al. 1991a) examined CSF somatostatin-like immunoactivity (SLI) and found lower levels than in aged matched controls. CSF SLI correlated significantly with CSF

5HIAA, suggesting an inter-relationship between somatostatin and serotonin systems in elderly depressed patients. No relationship was found, however, between SCF SLI levels and measures of thyroid function (Molchan et al. 1991b).

Growth hormone (GH) response to clonidine, a measure of α-2 noradrenergic receptor sensitivity, has been reported in several studies in younger patients (reviewed by Katona et al. 1987) to be blunted in depression. The test is, however, difficult to perform with elderly patients because of the risk of hypotension, and most studies have been restricted to patients under the age of 60 years. In such subjects, no clear relationship to age within depressed or control groups has been reported. A small study by Gilles et al. (1989) compared clonidine-induced GH secretion in elderly patients with major depressive disorder and with Alzheimer's disease. Very small responses were found in both groups, which did not differ significantly from each other. These results are, however, difficult to interpret in the absence of a control group and in the presence of another study showing no difference between patients suffering from Alzheimer's disease and age-matched controls (Peabody et al. 1986).

Both DST results and GH responses to clonidine may in part reflect age-related changes in neuroendocrine regulation. Schneider (1992) has suggested that normal aging may be associated with enhanced HPA axis activity due to age-associated neuronal degeneration in the hippocampus, which may in turn result from increased glucocorticoid levels. Veith and Raskind (1988) note that baseline GH secretion as well as GH response to provocative stimuli decrease gradually with age, probably because of age-related decreases in both size and number of growth hormone secretory cells in the pituitary.

PLATELET MARKERS

Because it is readily accessible and shares a number of membrane receptor and transport systems with the brain, the platelet has been extensively studied in depressed patients. Platelet markers most studied with respect to ageing and in particular to depression in old age have been monoamine-oxidase (MAO) levels, α-2 adrenoceptors and ^{3}H-imipramine (^{3}H-IMIP) binding sites (a measure thought to be related to the serotonin-specific active uptake site).

Platelet MAO levels increase with age, particularly in females, and have been reported to be increased in primary depression (Davidson et al. 1980). Alexopoulos et al. (1984a) reported higher platelet MAO activity in elderly female subjects with late first onset depression than in those whose illness began before the age of 55. Schneider et al. (1988), however, reported platelet MAO activity to be increased significantly in secondary depression compared with both control and primary depression groups of elderly subjects. Georgotas et al. (1986) found that, within elderly patients, elevated platelet MAO activity was associated with anhedonia, anxiety and a past history of depression. In a recent review of biological markers for depression in old age, Schneider (1992) concluded that platelet MAO activity was probably genetically determined and a marker for psychopathology in general rather than depression in particular. On this basis it is probably not aetiologically informative in the specific context of depression in old age.

Most, but not all studies of platelet α-2 adrenoceptors in younger subjects have reported an increase or no change in untreated depressed patients (Katona et al. 1987). Increased platelet α-2 adrenoceptors in elderly depressed patients compared with age-appropriate controls have been reported by Doyle et al. (1985). Age itself may, however, affect α-2 adrenoceptor numbers. Katona et al. (1989) reported a positive correlation between age and α-2 adrenoceptor number in control subjects but not depressed patients.

[3]H-IMIP binding has received rather more attention in the context of depression and aging. Several, but not all, studies in younger depressed patients, report a reduction in binding site number in depression (Theodorou et al. 1989). A positive correlation between H-IMIP binding and age in volunteers was reported by Schneider et al. (1985) and by Roy et al. (1987). Several other studies have, however, reported no such correlation (Braddock et al. 1986, Desmedt et al. 1987, Wagner et al. 1985). An early study by Suranyi-Cadotte et al. (1985) showed that ^{3}H-IMIP binding was significantly lower in elderly depressed patients than in a comparison roup with Alzheimer's disease. More recently, Schneider et al. (1988) reported that reduced platelet ^{3}H-IMIP binding was specific to primary depression (as opposed to depression secondary to medical illness) in elderly subjects, and Nemeroff et al. (1988) reported that the depression associated reduction in ^{3}H-IMIP binding density was more marked in older than in younger depressed subjects. Nemeroff's group (Husain et al. 1991) have also reported a significant inverse relationship in elderly depressed subjects between ^{3}H-IMIP binding density and frequency of MRI imaged subcortical hyperintensities.

EEG VARIABLES

Overall increases in waking EEG alpha amplitude have been consistently reported in depression (Schneider 1992). This finding holds true for elderly depressed patients, both when actively depressed (Brenner et al. 1986) and when recovered and drug free (Pollock and Schneider 1989). Within depressed elderly subjects, no differences in waking EEG variables between early and late first onset cases were reported by Heyman et al. (1991).

EEG variables measured during sleep show remarkably similar changes in depression and in normal aging (Veith and Raskind 1988). In particular, both depression and aging are associated with increased overall night-time wakefulness, and decreases in slow-wave sleep, total rapid eye movement (REM) sleep and rapid eye movement latency. It has indeed been claimed (Vogel et al. 1980) that suppression of REM sleep is the key mechanism underlying antidepressant action.

The Pittsburgh group have carried out several studies examining the use of EEG sleep variables in distinguishing elderly depressed and demented patients. Reynolds et al. (1988) found that four EEG sleep variables were altered in elderly depressed patients. REM latency was reduced, percentage REM sleep time and indeterminate non-REM sleep time were both increased and final waking was earlier. A discriminant function based on these variables was correct in 80 of cases in distinguishing depressed and demented elderly patients. Houck et al. (1991) had similar success with a discriminant function based on only three variables (sleep maintenance, percentage of REM sleep and percentage of indeterminate non-REM sleep). Reynolds et al. (1987) have also reported that elderly depressed patients undergoing sleep deprivation show less change in their sleep pattern than subjects with Alzheimer's disease or healthy controls.

NUTRITIONAL STATUS

Nutritional status has not been consistently reported as abnormal in elderly depressed subjects. Kivela et al. (1989) found no differences in haematological parameters or levels of folate or of vitamins C and B_{12} in elderly depressed subjects compared with age- and sex-matched controls. Similarly, Schlegel and Nieber (1985) reported plasma folate levels to be within the normal range in a group of elderly depressed patients with mild cognitive impairment, and found no correlation between the degree of cognitive impairment and the folic acid levels. Bell et al. (1990) suggested, however, that low blood levels of a number of vitamins, particularly those in the B complex, might be associated with poor neuropsychological test performance in such patients. In a subsequent intervention study (Bell et al. 1992), they found that oral administration of vitamin B complex was associated with significant improvement in vitamin status as well as non-significant trends towards greater improvement in scores on rating of depression and cognitive functioning. All but one of the subjects in their study had baseline vitamin levels within the normal range. Their findings suggest the possibility that clinical vitamin deficiencies may contribute towards depression and cognitive impairment in old age. It is, however, equally plausible that vitamin deficiency should result from poor nutrition secondary to depression-related loss of appetite and self-neglect.

CONCLUSIONS

Both social and biological factors appear to be of considerable importance in the aetiology of depression in old age. A positive family history (at least for those with early first onset), poverty and loneliness emerge as the most robust predisposing factors. Adverse life events (particularly bereavement) and deteriorating physical health appear to be the most powerful precipitants. Poor physical health also appears to be the single factor most important in impeding recovery from depression. On a more positive note, good social support (particularly in the form of an available confidant) and, perhaps, above average intelligence may protect elderly people from becoming depressed even in the face of adversity. Increasing age does not in itself appear to be associated with increasing risk of depression, though the parallel between age- and depression-associated neuroendocrine changes cannot be purely coincidental. The biological data (particularly from imaging studies) also offer some support for the notion that people who become depressed for the first time in late life may be depressed as the result of a neurodegenerative process. Further study is clearly needed to clarify inter-relationships between aetiologically relevant measures (such as MRI hyperintensities and platelet receptors). The use of magnetic resonance spectroscopy as a bridge between structural and functional imaging, and the development of SPET and PET techniques to measure the function of specific neurotransmitter systems have great potential in achieving such clarification.

REFERENCES

Abas MA, Sahakian BJ and Levy R (1990) Neuropsychological deficits and CT scan changes in elderly depressives. *Psychological Medicine* 20, 507–20.

Alexopoulos GS (1989) Biological abnormalities in late life depression. *Journal of Geriatric Psychiatry* 141, 25–34.

Alexopoulos GS, Lieberman KW and Young RC (1984a) Platelet MAO activity and age at onset of depression in elderly depressed women. *American Journal of Psychiatry* 141, 1276–8.

Alexopoulos GS, Young RC, Kocsis JH et al. (1984b) Dexamethasone suppression test in geriatric depression. *Biological Psychiatry* 19, 1567–71.

Alexopoulos GS, Young RC and Shindledecker RD (1992) Brain computed tomography findings in geriatric depression and primary degenerative dementia. *Biological Psychiatry* 31, 591–9.

Asnis GM, Sachar EJ, Halbreich V et al. (1981) Cortisol secretion in relation to age in major depression. *Psychosomatic Medicine* 43, 235–42.

Baldwin RC (1993) Late life depression and structural brain changes: a review of recent magnetic resonance imaging research. *International Journal of Geriatric Psychiatry* 8, 115–23.

Beats B and Levy R (1992) Imaging and affective disorders in the elderly. *Clinics in Geriatric Medicine* 8, 267–74.

Bell IR, Edman JD, Marby DW et al. (1990) Vitamin B_{12} and folate status in acute geropsychiatric inpatients: affective and cognitive characteristics of a vitamin non-deficient population. *Biological Psychiatry* 27, 125–37.

Bell IR, Edman JS, Morrow FD et al. (1992) Vitamin B_1, B_2, and B_6 augmentation of tricyclic antidepressant treatment in geriatric depression with cognitive dysfunction. *Journal of the American College of Nutrition* 11, 159–63.

Bench CJ, Friston KJ, Brown RG et al. (1992) The anatomy of melancholia—focal abnormalities of cerebral blood flow in major depression. *Psychological Medicine* 22, 607–15.

Blazer D, Birchett B, Service C and George LC (1991) The association of age and depression among the elderly: an epidemiologic exploration. *Journal of Gerontology* 46, M210–15.

Blazer D and Williams CD (1980) Epidemiology of dysphoria and depression in an elderly population. *American Journal of Psychiatry* 137, 439–44.

Braddock L, Cowen PJ, Elliott JM et al. (1986) Binding of yohimbine and imipramine to platelets in depressive illness. *Psychological Medicine* 16, 765–73.

Brenner RP, Ulrich RF, Spiker DG et al. (1986) Computerised EEG spectral analysis in elderly normal, demented and depressed subjects. *Electroencephalography and Clinical Neurophysiology* **64**, 483–92.

Brodaty H, Peters K, Boyce P et al. (1991) Age and depression. *Journal of Affective Disorders* **23**, 137–49.

Brown GW and Harris TO (1978) *Social Origins of Depression*. London, Tavistock.

Bruce ML and McNamara R (1992) Psychiatric status among the homebound elderly: an epidemiologic perspective. *Journal of the American Geriatric Society* **40**, 561–6.

Burke KC, Burke JD, Rae DS et al. (1991) Comparing age at onset of major depression and other psychiatric disorders by birth cohorts in five U.S. community populations. *Archives of General Psychiatry* **48**, 789–95.

Buschbaum M, Wu J, Delisi L et al. (1986) Frontal cortex and basal ganglia metabolic rates assessed by positron emission tomography with [18F] 2-deoxyglucose in affective illness. *Journal of Affective Disorders* **10**, 137–152.

Cadoret RJ and Widmer RB (1988) The development of depressive symptoms in elderly following onset of severe physical illness. *Journal of Family Practice* **27**, 71–6.

Carpiniello B, Carta, MG and Rudas N (1989) Depression among elderly people; a psychosocial study of urban and rural populations. *Acta Psychiatrica Scandinavica* **80**, 445–50.

Carroll BJ, Feinberg M, Greden JF et al. (1981) A specific laboratory test for the diagnosis of melancholia; standardisation, validation, and clinical utility. *Archives of General Psychiatry* **38**, 15–22.

Ciompi L (1969) Follow-up studies on the evolution of former neurotic and depressive states in old age: clinical and psychodynamic aspects. *Journal of Geriatric Psychiatry* **3**, 90–106.

Coffey CE, Figiel GS, Djang WT et al. (1988) Leukoencephalopathy in elderly depressed patients referred for ECT. *Biological Psychiatry* **24**, 143–161.

Coffey CE, Figiel GS, Djang WT et al. (1990) Subcortical hyperintensity on magnetic resonance imaging. A comparison of normal and depressed elderly subjects. *American Journal of Psychiatry* **147**, 187–9.

Davidson JRT, McLeod MN, Turnbull CD et al. (1980) Platelet monoamine oxidase activity and the classification of depression. *Archives of General Psychiatry* **37**, 771–3.

Davis KL, Davis BM, Mathe AA et al. (1984) Age and the dexamethasone suppression test in depression. *American Journal of Psychiatry* **141**, 872–4.

Dean A, Kolody B and Wood P (1990) Effects of social support from various sources on depression in elderly persons. *Journal of Health and Social Behaviour* **31**, 148–61.

Desmedt DH, Egrise D and Mendlewicz J (1987) Platelet imipramine binding sites in affective disorders and schizophrenia: influence of seasonal variation. *Journal of Affective Disorders* **12**, 192–8.

Dimond M, Lund DA and Caserta MS (1987) The role of social support in the first two years of bereavement in an elderly sample. *Gerontologist* **27**, 599–604.

Doyle MC, George AJ, Ravindran AV et al. (1985) Platelet α_2-adrenoreceptor binding in elderly depressed patients. *American Journal of Psychiatry* **142**, 1489–90.

Drinka TJK, Smith JC and Drinka PJ (1987) Correlates of depression and burden for informal caregivers of patients in a geriatric referral clinic. *Journal of the American Geriatric Society* **35**, 522–5.

Emerson JP, Burvill PW, Finlay-Jones R et al. (1989) Life events, life difficulties and confiding relationships in the depressed elderly. *British Journal of Psychiatry* **155**, 787–92.

Evans S and Katona CLE (1993) The epidemiology of depressive symptoms in elderly primary care attenders. *Dementia*, in press.

Figiel GS, Krishnan RRK, Deraiswamy PM et al. (1991) Subcortical hyperintensities on brain magnetic resonance imaging: a comparison between late age onset and early onset elderly depressed subjects. *Neurobiology of Aging* **26**, 245–7.

Gallagher D, Rose J, Rivera P et al. (1989) Prevalence of depression in family caregivers. *Gerontologist* **29**, 449–56.

Georgotas A, McCue RE, Kim OM et al. (1986) Dexamethasone suppression in dementia, depression and normal aging. *American Journal of Psychiatry* **143**, 452–6.

Gilles C, Ryckaert P, De Mol J et al. (1989) Clonidine-induced growth hormone secretion in elderly patients with senile dementia of the Alzheimer type and major depressive disorder. *Psychiatry Research* **27**, 277–86.

Gillis LS and Zabow A (1982) Dysphoria in the elderly. *South African Medical Journal* **62**, 410–13.

Greden JF, Flegel P, Haskett R et al. (1986) Age effects in serial hypothalamic–pituitary–adrenal monitoring. *Psychoneuroendocrinology* **11**, 195–204.

Heyman RA, Brenner RP, Reynolds CF et al. (1991) Age at initial onset of depression and wake EEG variables in the elderly. *Biological Psychiatry* **29**, 994–1000.

Hill DC, Thompson LW and Gallagher D (1988) The role of anticipatory bereavement in older women's adjustment to widowhood. *Gerontologist* **28**, 792–6.

Husain MM, Knight DL, Doraiswamy PM et al. (1991) Platelet [^{3}H]-imipramine binding and leukoencephalopathy in geriatric depression. *Biological Psychiatry* **29**, 665–70.

Husaini BA, Moore ST, Castor RS et al. (1991) Social density, stressors and depression: gender differences among the black elderly. *Journal of Gerontology* **46**, 236–42.

Houck PR, Reynolds CF, Mazumdar S et al. (1991) Receiver operating characteristic analysis for validating EEG sleep discrimination of elderly depressed and demented paients. *Journal of Geriatric Psychiatry and Neurology* **4**, 30–3.

Jacoby RJ and Levy R (1980) Computed tomography in the elderly: affective disorder. *British Journal of Psychiatry* **136**, 270–5.

Jacoby RJ, Levy R and Bird JM (1981) Computed tomography and the outcome of affective disorder; a follow-up study of elderly patients. *British Journal of Psychiatry* **139**, 288–92.

Katona CLE, Theodorou AE, Davies SL et al. (1989) ^{3}H Yohimbine binding to platelet α_2-adrenoceptors in depression. *Journal of Affective Disorders* **17**, 219–28.

Katona CLE, Theodorou AE and Horton RW (1987) α_2-adrenoceptors in depression. *Psychiatric Developments* **2**, 129–49.

Kennedy GJ, Kelman HR, Thomas C et al. (1989) Hierarchy of characteristics associated with depressive symptoms in an urban elderly sample. *American Journal of Psychiatry* **146**, 220–5.

Kennedy GJ, Kelman HR, Thomas C et al. (1990) The emergence of depressive symptoms in late life: the importance of declining health and increasing disability. *Journal of Community Health* **15**, 93–104.

Kivela S-L and Pahkala K (1991) Relationships between health behaviour and depression in the aged. *Aging* **3**, 153–9.

Kivela S-L, Pahkala K and Eronen A (1989) Depression in the aged: relation to folate and vitamins C and B$_{12}$. *Biological Psychiatry* **26**, 210–13.

Lewinsohn PR, Seeley JR and Fischer SA (1991) Age and depression: unique and shared effects. *Psychology and Aging* **6**, 247–60.

Lewis DA, Pfohl B, Schlechte J et al. (1984) Influence of age on the cortisol response to dexamethasone. *Psychiatry Research* **13**, 213–20.

Linn MW, Hunter K and Harris R (1980) Symptoms of depression and recent life events in the community elderly. *Journal of Clinical Psychology* **36**, 675–82.

Loosen PT, Marciniak R and Thadani K (1987) TRH-induced TSH response in healthy volunteers: relationship to psychiatric history. *American Journal of Psychiatry* **144**, 455–9.

Maes M, Minner B, Suy E et al. (1991) Cortisol escape from suppression by dexamethasone during depression is strongly predicted by basal cortisol hypersecretion and increasing age combined. *Psychoneuroendrocrinology* **16**, 295–310.

Molchan SE, Hill JL, Mellow AM et al. (1990) The dexamethasone suppression test in Alzheimer's disease and major depression: relationship to dementia severity, depression and CSF monoamines. *International Psychogeriatrics* 2, 99–122.

Molchan SE, Lawlor BA, Hill JL et al. (1991a) CSF monoamine metabolites and somatostatin in Alzheimer's disease and major depression. *Biological Psychiatry* 29, 1110–18.

Molchan SE, Lawlor BA, Hill JL et al. (1991b) The TRH stimulation test in Alzheimer's disease and major depression. *Biological Psychiatry* 30, 567–76.

Murphy E (1982) Social origins of deession in old age. *British Journal of Psychiatry* 141, 135–42.

Murrell SA, Meeks S and Walker J (1991) Protective functions of health and self-esteem against depression in older adults facing illness or bereavement. *Psychology and Aging* 6, 352–60.

Nemeroff CR, Knight DL, Krishnan RR et al. (1988) Marked reductions in the number of platelet tritiated imipramine binding sites in geriatric depression. *Archives of General Psychiatry* 45, 919–23.

Oxman TE, Berkman LF, Kasl S et al. (1992) Social support and depressive symptoms in the elderly. *American Journal of Epidemiology* 135, 356–68.

Pahkala K, Kivela S-L and Laippala P (1991) Social and environmental factors and major depression in old age. *Zeitschrift für Gerontologie* 24, 17–23.

Peabody CA, Minkoff JR, Davies HD et al. (1986) Thyrotropin releasing hormone test and Alzheimer's disease. *Biological Psychiatry* 21, 553–6.

Pearlson GD, Rabins PV, Kim WS et al. (1989) Structural brain CT changes and cognitive deficits in elderly depressives with and without reversible dementia ('pseudodementia'). *Psychological Medicine* 19, 573–84.

Phillips CJ and Henderson AS (1991) The prevalence of depression among Australian nursing home residents; results using draft ICD10 and DSMIII R criteria. *Psychological Medicine* 21, 739–48.

Pollock VE and Schneider LS (1989) Topographic electroencephalographic alpha in recoved depressed elderly. *Journal of Abnormal Psychology* 98, 268–73.

Post F and Shulman K (1985) New views on old age affective disorders. In Arie T (ed.) *Recent Developments in Psychogeriatrics*. London, Churchill Livingstone.

Pruchno RA and Resch NL (1989) Husbands and wives as caregivers: antecedents of depression and burden. *Gerontologist* 29, 159–65.

Rabins PV, Pearlson GD, Aylward E (1991) Cortical magnetic resonance imaging changes in elderly patients with major depression. *American Journal of Psychiatry* 148, 617–20.

Reynolds CF, Kupfer DJ, Hoch CC et al. (1987) Sleep deprivation as probe in the elderly. *Archives of General Psychiatry* 44, 982–91.

Reynolds CF, Kupfer DJ, Houck PR et al. (1988) Reliable discrimination of elderly depressed and demented patients by electroencephalographic sleep data. *Archives of General Psychiatry* 45, 258–64.

Rotenberg KJ and Hamel J (1988) Social interaction and depression in elderly individuals. *International Journal of Aging and Human Development* 27(A), 305–18.

Roy A, Everett D, Pickar D and Paul SM (1987) Platelet tritiated imipramine binding and serotonin uptake in depressed patients and controls. Relationship to plasma cortisol before and after dexamethasone administration. *Archives of General Psychiatry* 44, 320–7.

Russell DW and Cutrona CE (1991) Social support, stress and depressive symptoms among the elderly: test of a process model. *Psychology and Aging* 6, 190–201.

Sackheim HA, Prohovnik I, Moeller JR et al. (1990) Regional cerebral blood flow in mood disorders. I. Comparison of major depressives and normal controls at rest. *Archives of General Psychiatry* 47, 60–70.

Saunders PA, Copeland JR, Dewey ME et al. (1991) Heavy drinking as a risk factor for depression and dementia in elderly men: findings from the Liverpool Longitudinal Community Study. *British Journal of Psychiatry* 159, 213–16.

Schlegel S and Nieber D (1985) Folic acid and cognition in the elderly depressed. *Biological Psychiatry* 25, 976–7.

Schneider LS (1992) Psychobiologic features of geriatric affective disorder. *Clinics in Geriatric Medicine* 8, 253–65.

Schneider LS, Leverson JA and Sloane RB (1985) Platelet ^{3}H-imipramine binding in depressed elderly patients. *Biological Psychiatry* 20, 1232–4.

Schneider LS, Severson JA, Sloane RB et al. (1988) Decreased platelet ^{3}H-imipramine binding in primary major depression compared with depression secondary to medical illness in elderly outpatients. *Journal of Affective Disorders* 15, 195–200.

Schulz R and Williamson GM (1991) A 2-year longitudinal study of depression among Alzheimer's caregivers. *Psychology and Aging* 6, 569–78.

Shields CG (1992) Family interaction and caregivers of Alzheimer's disease patients: correlates of depression. *Family Process* 31, 19–33.

Shulman KI, Tohen M and Satlin A (1992) Mania revisited. In Arie T (ed.) *Recent Advances in Psychogeriatrics*. London, Churchill Livingstone.

Siegel B, Gurevich D and Oxenkrug F (1989) Cognitive impairment and cortisol resistance to dexamethasone sppression in elderly depression. *Biological Psychiatry* 25, 229–34.

Silfverskiold P and Risberg J (1989) Regional cerebral blood flow in depression and mania. *Archives of General Psychiatry* 46, 253–9.

Smallegan M (1989) Level of depressive symptoms and life stresses for culturally diverse older adults. *The Gerontologist* 29, 45–50.

Stephenson-Cino P, Steiner M, Kramer L et al. (1992) Depression in elderly persons and its correlates in family practice: a Canadian study. *Psychological Reports* 70, 359–68.

Suranyi-Cadotte, BE, Gauthier S, Lafaille F et al. (1985) Platelet ^{3}H-imipramine binding distinguishes depression from Alzheimer dementia. *Life Sciences* 37, 2305–11.

Theodorou AE, Katona CLE, Davies SL et al. (1989) ^{3}H-imipramine binding to freshly prepared platelet membranes in depression. *Psychiatry Research* 29, 87–103.

Tourigny-Rivard MF, Raskind M and Rivard D (1981) The dexamethasone suppression test in an elderly population. *Biological Psychiatry* 16, 1177–84.

Veith RC and Raskind MA (1988) The neurobiology of aging: does it predispose to depression? *Neurobiology of Aging* 9, 101–17.

Vogel GWF, Vogel RS, McAbee RS and Thurmond AJ (1980) Improvement of depression REM sleep deprivation. *Archives of General Psychiatry* 37, 247–53.

Wagner A, Aberg-Wistedt A, Asberg M et al. (1985) Lower ^{3}H-imipramine binding in platelets from untreated depressed patients compared to healthy controls. *Psychiatry Research* 16, 131–9.

Warshaw MG, Klerman GL and Lavori PW (1991) The use of conditional probabilities to examine age–period–cohort data: further evidence for a period effect in major depessive disorder. *Journal of Affective Disorders* 23, 119–29.

Weiner MF, Davis BM, Mohs RC et al. (1987) Influence of age and relative weight on cortisol suppression in normal subjects. *American Journal of Psychiatry* 144, 646–9.

Zisook S, Shuchter SR and Lyons LE (1987) Predictors of psychological reactions during the early stages of widowhood. *Psychiatric Clinics of North America* 10, 355–68.

5 Depression and Physical Illness in Old Age

INTRODUCTION

Elderly patients with serious physical illness often have symptoms of depression (Blazer 1980). At times, such reactions may be appropriate and require only supportive care, but in many cases symptoms persist for an extended period and interfere with social functioning or even basic self-care. Particular care must be taken to distinguish clinical depression from the mere presence of one or more depressive symptoms. Links between depression and specific physical conditions such as cerebrovascular disease and some endocrine disorders have been described. If depression is not recognised and treated it may have an impact on recovery from the physical illness, leading to extended hospital stays with increased mortality. Awareness of depression by the responsible physician and its effective management may therefore make a considerable contribution to improving patient care. The epidemiology and management of depression coexisting with physical illness will be considered below in the specific clinical contexts in which it occurs.

HOSPITAL INPATIENTS

Although the reported prevalence of depression in elderly medical inpatients has varied between 10% and 45% (Rapp et al. 1988b), several studies have reached a consensus of around 15% (see Table 5.1). Ramsay et al. (1991) used the depression and organic brain syndrome scales from the SHORT-CARE (Gurland et al. 1984; see also Chapter 2) to identify depressive symptomatology in a consecutive series of 119 elderly acute medical patients. Only 88 (74%) could complete the depression interview and, of those, 35 (29% of the total) had depressive symptoms and 9 (8%) a diagnosis of depression. The prevalence of significant depressive symptomatology was similar (48%) in chronic geriatric admissions (Shah et al. 1992).

Overall, the rate for affective disorder in elderly medical inpatients appears similar to that in comparable younger groups (Mayou and Hawton 1986), although Feldman et al. (1987) carried out a systematic comparison and found a relatively lower prevalence in their elderly subsample of inpatients. Koenig et al. (1991), in a study of older (age > 70) and younger men admitted to the medical

Table 5.1   Acute hospital prevalence of depression

Study	Prevalence (%)	Diagnostic criteria	Sample size	Population
Bergmann and Eastham (1974)	19	Clinical	100	Medical
Cheah et al. (1980)	37	DSM III	143	Medical
Millar (1981)	11	Clinical	100	Surgical
Kitchell et al. (1982)	45	DSM III	42	Medical
Cooper (1987)	41	CASE/CSI	626	DGH
Feldman et al. (1987)	10	PSE/CATEGO	133	Medical
Johnston et al. (1987)	17	GHQ	168	DGH
Rapp et al. (1988b)	15	RDC	150	Medical
Koenig et al. (1988a)	12	DSM III	130	Medical
O'Riordan (1989)	23	DSM III	111	Medical
Harper et al. (1990)	59 (major)	RDC	247	Geriatric
Lazaro et al. (1991)	21	DSM IIIR	112	Medical and surgical
Rapp et al. (1991)	16	RDC	102	Medical
Ramsay et al. (1991)	29 (symptoms) 8 (diagnosed)	SHORT-CARE	119	Geriatric
Koenig et al. (1991)	13 (major) 29 (minor)	DSM IIIR	332	Male medical

wards of a veterans' hospital, found a similar overall prevalence of depression, using DSM IIIR (American Psychiatric Association 1987) criteria, in the two groups. Major depression was, however, commoner in younger patients and minor depression in the older group. As discussed in Chapter 1, this may reflect, at least in part, age-related differences in the performance of diagnostic criteria.

Some of these differences in prevalence rates for depression may be explained on methodological grounds (Rodin and Voshart 1986). Studies vary in patient inclusion and exclusion criteria, in choice of diagnostic categories, and (in the absence, as discussed in Chapter 2, of generally accepted screening instruments) in the methods used to detect depression. Harper et al. (1990) used a variety of screening instruments and found that all underdetected both major and, to a greater extent, minor depression as identified using Research Diagnostic Criteria (RDC; Spitzer and Endicott 1978). The strikingly high overall rate of depression in their sample was however due, in their view, to the fact that the patients included were 'representative of a select group of patients with a likely high base rate of depression. That is, they were identified by family members or their physicians as showing an unexplained deterioration in their functioning of a magnitude to warrant medical evaluation and/or intervention.' Feldman et al. (1987), in contrast, reported a much lower rate of depression (10%) in acute medical admissions aged 70 and over. This probably reflects their use of the Present State Examination (PSE; Wing et al. 1974), which has relatively narrow criteria for diagnosing depression and does not take into account the different patterns of clinical features found in elderly depressed patients.

Another difficulty clinicians face in recognising cases of depression in the medically ill elderly is that it may present covertly, in particular with psychosomatic symptoms or with hypochondriasis, which may lead to confusion with the coexisting physical illness. Cavanaugh et al. (1983) suggest that the diagnosis should be borne in mind particularly when there is dysphoria or anhedonia which does not respond to treatment of the underlying medical condition. In a study of 60 elderly patients in a general hospital referred for psychiatric assessment (Kua 1987), 41% had a depressive illness.

Depression may be an important aetiological factor contributing to 'unexplained deterioration in functioning'. The study by Harper et al. (1990) referred to earlier found that, among 247 such patients, depression had a very high prevalence: using RDC criteria, 59% of the patients suffered from major depression and 21 from minor depression. There may also be confusion with cognitive impairment, leading to incorrect diagnoses of dementia (Marsden and Harrison 1972).

In view of this, it is perhaps not surprising that the rate of detection of depression by hospital physicians is low: Rapp et al. (1988a) found only 8.7% of depressed patients were identified by house staff (76). In a further study, Rapp and Davis (1989) evaluated medical residents' knowledge and revealed that although the staff considered detection and treatment of co-morbid depression important, they knew few of the diagnostic criteria and relevant aetiological factors, rarely screened their patients for depression and viewed available treatments as only marginally efficacious. Koenig et al. (1988b) found a similarly low rate of documentation of depressive symptoms (20%) by house staff, which increased to only 27% after they had been informed of the possibility of major depression. Only half the latter group were given antidepressant therapy. While this low detection rate and even lower treatment rate might indicate a lack of sensitivity of clinicians to depression in this population, the physicians' reluctance to use antidepressants may be partly explained by the observation that 87% of the depressed patients had relative or absolute contraindications to antidepressants (Koenig et al. 1988b).

Few studies have examined the natural history of depression in elderly medical inpatients. We have reported depression to be persistent in the majority of both acute and continuing-care elderly medical patients followed up at one year, but not to be associated with increased mortality (Finch et al. 1991; Shah et al. 1992). Very similar findings of persistence of depression (associated with very low rates of treatment) have been reported by Rapp et al. (1991). Harris et al. (1988) assessed medical rehabilitation patients on admission and at discharge, and found significant correlations between improvement in depression rating and improvement in level of dependency. All patients whose mood improved also improved in level of physical functioning; such functional improvement was seen in only 25% of those who remained depressed. There was a trend, which just failed to reach statistical significance, for improvement in depression to be associated with its detection by medical staff and with the administration of antidepressants.

LIAISON REFERRALS

Kua (1987) found depression to be the most frequent diagnosis (41.6%) among elderly medical patients referred to psychiatrists, while Mainprize and Rodin (1987) found it to be second to dementia (17% vs 51%). Overall, however, psychiatric referral rate is low in elderly medical patients in comparison with younger patients (Folks and Ford 1985). Referral is more likely in elderly women than elderly men and comes more frequently from some specialities, including internal medicine and neurology than, for example, surgery. Pauser et al. (1987) found that the establishment of a liaison service increased the rate of referrals, and that knowledge by the physicians of a patient's past psychiatric history also increased the likelihood that he or she would be referred to the liaison psychiatry service.

SPECIFIC MEDICAL CONDITIONS

STROKE (see Table 5.2)

The review by Koenig and Studenski (1988) found that 30–65% of individuals were depressed in the year following a stroke. Starkstein and Robinson (1989) made a similar estimate of its prevalence as between 30% and 50%. Wade et al. (1987), in a community study of 976 patients, found that 25–30% of them were depressed on at least one of three occasions in the year following a stroke. Eastwood et al. (1989) found 10% of 87 stroke inpatients to have major depression and a further 50% minor depression. These studies confirmed earlier work by Folstein et al. (1977), who found that 45% of stroke patients were depressed compared with 10% of orthopaedic patients. In contrast to this, House et al. (1991) found only 12% of a series of 128 patients identified in the community and seen one month after their stroke to be PSE 'cases' of depression. This was, however, significantly higher than the rate of 7.5% found in matched community controls. The relatively low prevalence found in this study probably reflects the reduced risk of depression encountered by patients able to be cared for at home after their stroke compared with those needing hospitalisation.

Depression associated with stroke is often chronic. Wade et al. (1987) found that 50% of their depressed patients remained so for over a year. A similar rate of chronicity was identified by Eastwood et al. (1989) at four months. A number of risk factors have been suggested for post-stroke depression. Wade et al. (1987) found that depression was associated with loss of independence, low activity level and poor mobility, as did the majority of reports (including their own) reviewed by Schubert et al. (1992), though the important study by Starkstein and Robinson

Table 5.2 Prevalence of depression in stroke patients

Study	Prevalence (%)	Diagnostic criteria	Sample
Starkstein and Robinson (1989)	30–50	Review	
Koenig and Studenski (1988)	30–65	Review	
Eastwood et al. (1989)	50 (10 major, 40 minor)	RDC (SADS)	In-patient
Wade et al. (1987)	25–30	Wakefield Depression Inventory	Community
Robinson and Price (1982)	41	GHQ (Zung, HDRS, PSE)	Outpatient rehab. clinic
Robinson and Szetela (1981)	60	Zung, HDRS	Inpatient (+ control)
Folstein et al. (1977)	45	HDRS	Inpatient (+ control)
House et al. (1991)	12	PSE	Community (+ control)

(1989) failed to replicate this. Many studies have investigated the relationship between the anatomical location of the stroke and the severity of depression. There seems to be some agreement that depression may be more common in those with left hemisphere lesions, particularly those in the left frontal pole (East wood et al. 1989; Lipsey et al. 1984; Robinson and Szetela 1981). A recent study of male stroke victims with a mean age of 66 (Stern and Bachman 1991) suggests that the relationship between lesion location and mood disturbance may be more complex than previously thought, with a three-way interaction being found between likelihood of dysphoric mood on the one hand and right/left, dorsal/ventral and frontal/non-frontal lesion position on the other.

It has been suggested that neuroendocrine abnormalities may underlie the development of post-stroke depression. In this regard the dexamethasone suppression test (DST) has been intensively investigated, since (as discussed in Chapter 4) it may have particularly high sensitivity and specificity for depression in old age. Most studies suggest, however, that the DST does not discriminate usefully between depressed and non-depressed stroke patients (Grober et al. 1991).

The problem of detecting depression may be particularly severe in stroke patients. This is most evident in the context of aphasia (Koenig and Studenski 1988) or acute concurrent medical illness (Eastwood et al. 1989). It may also be difficult to decide clinically as to the relative contribution of depression and of true post-stroke brain damage in patients whose cooperation with physiotherapy and general rehabilitation appears disproportionately poor. The difficulties involved in using rating scales to detect depression in stroke patients is well reviewed by House et al. (1989).

OTHER CEREBRAL LESIONS

There has been little attention paid to the association between depression and other focal brain lesions. Robinson and Szetela (1981) compared patients with left hemisphere lesions following stroke and trauma. They found an incidence of only 20% for depression in the trauma patients compared with 60% in stroke patients. Depression as well as many other psychiatric problems is found in patients with cerebral tumours (Lishman 1987), but there have been no specific studies looking at the risk of this in the elderly.

CANCER

Cancer is predominantly a disease of the elderly and seems to be associated with substantial depression. This may be especially so with carcinoma of the pancreas (Fras et al. 1968). Barraclough (1971) in his classic study of suicide in the elderly found a significant excess of terminal malignancies (often undiagnosed before death) compared with matched controls dying through accidental death (see Chapter 6). Whitlock (1978) also found an excess of tumours in a somewhat younger group of suicides.

The inter-relationship between malignancy and depression is complex. As well as being an understandable reaction to learning of a diagnosis of cancer, and a non-metastatic complication of malignant disease in its own right, depression may also be a reflection of other non-metastatic complications. In support of the latter hypothesis, Weizman et al. (1979) studied 12 patients with a mean age of 60 who had hypercalcaemia associated with a neoplasm. Seven had symptoms of psychiatric disturbance, predominantly either acute confusional states or depression. These symptoms resolved when the calcium levels had returned to normal. Finally, an existing depressive illness may, by altering immune responsiveness, predispose patients to the subsequent development of malignancy (Schliefer et al. 1985).

PARKINSON'S DISEASE

The association between Parkinson's disease (PD) and depression in the elderly is well documented (Mindham 1970). More recent studies have confirmed this association and attempted to describe it more fully. Robins (1976) studied 45 patients with a mean age of 69 and compared them with chronically disabled controls. He found an increased prevalence of depression in PD which was unaffected by the degree of physical disability experienced by the patients. Mayeux et al. (1981) confirmed the high prevalence of depression in PD and found a possible association with mild intellectual impairment. A further study by Mayeux et al. (1986) suggests that depression in PD may be associated with reduced cerebrospinal fluid levels of the serotonin metabolite 5-hydroxyindoleacetic acid. Huber et al. (1988) suggested that PD patients with significant tremor had less depression than those with bradykinesia. In a retrospective case-note study of a large, predominantly elderly (mean age 71) sample of patients with PD, Dooneief et al. (1992) found the prevalence of depression (using DSM IIIR criteria) to be as high as 47%, with an annual incidence of 1.9%. Surprisingly, no significant associations were found between depression and PD variables such as age at onset and duration of PD, duration of treatment with L-dopa, or degree of disability.

ENDOCRINE AND METABOLIC DISORDERS

High levels of circulating glucocorticoid can cause depression, which was a common feature in Cushing's (1932) description of his eponymous syndrome. Cohen (1980) studied a group of 29 patients of mixed ages with Cushing's syndrome and found that 86% were depressed. Depression may also occur in the context of therapeutic administration of glucocorticoids (Bell 1991), though this has not been studied specifically in the elderly. The low levels of circulating glucocorticoid that constitute Addison's disease are also associated with depression, although it tends to be a disease found in early middle age, only rarely affecting the elderly (Lishman 1987).

Hypothyroidism presents relatively frequently in old age and its clinical features overlap considerably with those of depression. Occasionally a pure depressive syndrome is seen. Sappy et al. (1987) suggested a relationship between sick euthyroid syndrome (in which thyroxine levels remain in the normal range but thyroid stimulating hormone is raised) and neurotic depression in the elderly. Drinka and Voeks (1988), however, failed to replicate this. Hyperthyroidism is less common in the elderly but may occasionally be associated with depression, although it is more commonly found in association with anxiety.

Hyperparathyroidism is a rare but significant cause of depression which may be found in the elderly. Peterson (1968) found 36% of a series of patients to have some affective changes although he fails to mention their ages. Cooper and Schapira (1973) described a 64-year-old woman whose hyperparathyroidism was complicated by depression. The depression resolved when the hyperparathyroidism was treated and the calcium returned to normal.

RELATIONSHIP BETWEEN PHYSICAL ILLNESS AND DEPRESSION

Risk factors for depression within the physically ill elderly appear similar to those (discussed in Chapter 4) for depression in old age as a whole. Increasing severity of physical disorder increases the risk of depression in the medically ill elderly

(Koenig et al. 1988a, 1991; Rapp et al. 1988b). Amongst elderly elective surgical patients, Millar (1981) noted developing or persisting depression to be associated with post-operative medical complications. Coexisting cognitive dysfunction and low education (Koenig et al. 1988c), lack of a spouse or support system (Koenig et al. 1991; Stewart 1991) and degree of functional disability (Koenig et al. 1991), as well as a past psychiatric history (Koenig et al. 1988c), are also associated with an increased rate of depression.

As far as the overall and, as discussed above, well-established association between physical illness and depression is concerned, the aetiological link is not at all clear. Eastwood and Corbin (1986) have suggested four hypotheses to explain it.

1. The observed relationship may be coincidental and reflect an increased incidence and prevalence of both pathologies. Epidemiological studies of depression do not support this since the prevalence of depression changes little between middle and old age (see Chapter 3).
2. Physical illness may produce depression. This is likely for some specific conditions such as stroke, but no specific aetiological mechanisms have been put forward and no studies have measured pre-morbid psychiatric function.
3. Depression may produce physical illness through some effect on physiological functioning. Parkes et al. (1969) described increased deaths from myocardial infarction among widows during the six months following the death of their spouse, but pointed out that many of these men did have preexisting heart disease.
4. Physical and psychiatric morbidity may interact in response to chronic disease with pre-morbid personality as an important mediating variable.

There is as yet insufficient evidence to provide clear-cut support for these hypotheses or, indeed, to refute them.

EFFECT OF DEPRESSION ON THE OUTCOME OF PHYSICAL ILLNESS

Koenig et al. (1989c) found that medically ill patients with major depression consumed more health care resources as well as experiencing greater mortality. Other studies (reviewed by Gurland et al. 1988) have found that affective disorders may prolong the length of hospital stay. A problem with most of the above studies is the lack of allowance made for severity of physical illness in assessing the effect of co-morbid depression on service use. We did not find depression in acute geriatric admissions to be associated with increased bed occupancy, once allowance had been made for severity of physical illness (Ramsay et al. 1991). In contrast, Koenig et al. (1989c) demonstrated in a similar sample that depression *was* associated with increased use of health care resources independent of the severity of physical illness, in keeping with our own findings in elderly acute hip fracture patients (Shamash et al. 1992).

PROGNOSIS OF DEPRESSION IN THE PHYSICALLY ILL ELDERLY

The prognosis for depression in the physically ill may be worse than in the physically well. Murphy (1983) found that chronic health problems and acute new physical illness predicted poor outcome, and at four-year follow-upr mortality within the subjects depressed at baseline was much greater among those with major health problems (Murphy et al. 1988). The results suggested that although physical health contributed to the excess mortality as compared with age- and sex-matched controls, depression itself had an independent effect. Baldwin and Jolley (1986) report similar findings; 91% of patients experiencing a lasting recovery from depression had no active physical pathology on presentation, while 71% of those who remained continuously depressed had at least one active physical health problem on admission. In keeping with this, Harris et al. (1988) found that in a group of 30 patients depression was associated with poor physical rehabilitation. By contrast, however, Burvill et al. (1991) found no association between acute or chronic physical illness and depression.

TREATMENT

Therapeutic nihilism is a particular trap in elderly medical patients with coexisting depression. Clinicians should be alert to contraindications to antidepressants and to the development of side-effects. According to Katz et al. (1990) such drug side-effects are more prevalent in the frail elderly and for this reason a lower dose of tricyclic antidepressants may be necessary. Particular care is also needed due to the danger of toxic effects in overdose (Montgomery 1990).

Given the ameliorating effect of good-quality social support (Arling 1987), the setting in which care is given is also important. Vogel and Kroessler (1987) suggest there may be three alternatives for the inpatient treatment of elderly patients with depression and coexisting medical illness. They may be treated under medical services with psychiatric consultation and liaison; they may be transferred to a traditional psychiatric unit with medical consultation; or they can be managed in a specialised joint care setting—the medical psychiatric unit. Cole et al.(1991) have attempted to evaluate the effectiveness of geriatric psychiatry consultation in a group of referrals unselected by psychiatric diagnosis, and reported a non-significant trend towards benefit in the active intervention group. Unfortunately, only five patients in this group had a diagnosis of depression, so that meaningful conclusions about efficacy cannot be drawn.

The clinical challenge of controlled trials of antidepressant treatment in this population is considerable. This is epitomised in the report by Koenig et al. (1989a). They attempted a trial of nortriptyline against placebo in elderly patients admitted to the medical wards of a VA hospital. Though 964 were evaluated, only 773 were cognitively well enough preserved to allow GDS screening. Eighty-one scored positive for depression, and 63 of them were further evaluated by a psychiatrist. Forty-one were found to have DSM III major depressive episode, but 14 of them had already been treated with antidepressants, 15 had medical contraindications to their use and five refused. Of seven subjects randomised, four dropped out. Three completed the study, two on placebo and one on nortriptyline.

A number of small trials have, however, been successfully completed. Lipsey et al. (1984) have demonstrated the efficacy of nortriptyline in the treatment of post-stroke depression in a double-blind study of 34 patients with a mean age around 60. Patients who were successfully treated had serum nortriptyline levels in the conventional therapeutic range. It should be noted, however that only 14 patients were on active treatment, and of these three developed antidepressant-related acute confusional states. Reding et al. (1986) reported that trazodone showed a non-significant trend towards benefit when compared with placebo in stroke patients. Their findings are, however, difficult to interpret since not all subjects entered in the trial were clinically depressed and the main outcome measure was change in level of dependency rather than alleviation of depression. Schifano et al. (1990) compared the efficacy of mianserin and maprotiline in 48 elderly physically ill subjects with DSM IIIR major depression or (in four cases) dysthymia. Thirty-five completed the trial, with mianserin showing significant superiority in terms of GDS scores. Only 40% of subjects in each group, however, were improved or very much improved in terms of clinical global impression.

Despite the relative lack of controlled-trial evidence demonstrating the efficacy of specific treatments for depression in physically ill elderly patients, such treatment is nonetheless often necessary in clinical practice. Close links between geriatrician and psychiatrist are important to ensure that the possibility of co-morbid depression is considered in the initial assessment and subsequent care of elderly patients admitted to acute or chronic hospital beds. Treatment should be considered particularly in patients with prominent neurovegetative symptoms (particularly retardation, poor appetite and poor food and fluid intake) unexplained by their physical condition. Other 'pointers' to initiate treatment of depression include the expression of suicidal thoughts or intent, and depressive symptoms that are persistent, intense or impair social functioning. Patients who become depressed while undergoing medical treatment may become intolerant of levels of pain or disability that they were previously able to withstand without complaint. The possibility of depression should also be considered in patients whose medical problems fail to respond to apparently appropriate and usually effective treatment.

Systematic trials of antidepressants with better side-effect profiles and fewer medical contraindications are clearly needed in this population who, from the point of view of the pharmaceutical companies involved, represent a considerable potential market. Vogel and Kroessler (1987) suggest that MAOIs may be a safer option among elderly depressed patients and, indeed, many elderly patients who do not respond to tricylics will respond favourably to one of the MAOIs. Lithium augmentation, despite the relatively high risk of toxicity it carries in the frail elderly, has been specifically reported to be beneficial in physically ill elderly patients with refractory depression (Kushnir 1986).

Benbow (1989), reviewing the role of electroconvulsive therapy in the treatment of depressive illness in old age, indicated that it was safe and efficacious even if there was concomitant serious medical illness. Gaspar and Samarasinghe (1982) found that 10 of their sample of 33 elderly medical inpatients had major, and 15 minor, risk factors on the basis of a physical examination, past and present history, and investigations, but even in the major risk factor group, ECT appeared very safe and no patient died of anaesthetic or ECT complications. Cardiovascular problems do, however, remain a concern for elderly patients receiving ECT. For example, among a group of 42 patients with preexisting cardiac disease, 70% developed signs of ischaemia or an arrhythmia during a course of ECT, which in some cases were potentially life threatening (Gerring and Shields 1982). All such complications occurred in patients aged over 50 and the majority were over 60.

ECT has also been useful in other groups, such as in patients on anticoagulant therapy (Loo et al. 1985) and those with Parkinson's disease (Atre-Vaidya and Jampala 1988). In the latter case, it may be of particular benefit as such patients often respond poorly and experience worsening of their Parkinsonian symptoms with drug treatment. ECT may, in contrast, actually improve Parkinsonian symptoms (Ward et al. 1980).

CONCLUSIONS

The prevalence of depression in the physically ill elderly is clearly high. This is of considerably more than mere academic interest, since there are strong suggestions that the coexistence of depression and physical morbidity in old age worsens the prognosis of both. Routine screening for depression in geriatric patients is feasible and offers significant improvement over routine detection by junior medical staff. There are, however, several questions which remain unanswered. The aetiology and mechanism of the association between physical illness and depression are unknown and there has been a dearth of studies assessing the feasibility and utility of specific treatments for depression in the elderly physically ill.

REFERENCES

American Psychiatric Association (1987) *Diagnostic and Statistical Manual of Mental Disorders* (3rd edn, revised). Washington, American Psychiatric Association.
Arling G (1987) Strain, social support, and distress in old age. *Journal of Gerontology* **42**, 107–13.

Atre-Vaidya N and Jampala BC (1988) Electroconvulsive therapy in Parkinsonism with affective disorder. *British Journal of Psychiatry* **152**, 55–8.

Baldwin RC and Jolley DJ (1986) The prognosis of depression in old age. *British Journal of Psychiatry* **149**, 574–83.

Barraclough BM (1971) Suicide in the elderly. In Kay SWK and Walk AA (eds) *Recent Developments in Psychogeriatrics* (*British Journal of Psychiatry* special publications). Ashford, Headley Bros.

Bell G (1991) Steroid-induced psychiatric disorders. *Nordic Journal of Psychiatry* **45**, 437–41.

Benbow SM (1989) The role of electroconvulsive therapy in the treatment of depressive illness in old age. *British Journal of Psychiatry* **155**, 147–52.

Bergmann K and Eastham EJ (1974) Psychogeriatric ascertainment and assessment for treatment in an acute medical ward setting. *Age and Ageing* **3**, 174–88.

Blazer D (1980) The diagnosis of depression in the elderly. *Journal of the American Geriatrics Society* **28**, 52–8.

Burvill PW, Hall WD, Stampfer HG et al. (1991) The prognosis of depression in old age. *British Journal of Psychiatry* **158**, 64–71.

Cavanaugh S, Clark DC and Gibbons RD (1983) Diagnosing depression in the hospitalized medically ill. *Psychosomatics* **24**, 809–13.

Cheah KC and Beard OW (1980) Psychiatric findings in the population of a geriatric evaluation unit: implications. *Journal of the American Geriatrics Society* **28**, 153–6.

Cohen SI (1980) Cushing's syndrome: a psychiatric study of 29 patients *British Journal of Psychiatry* **136**, 120–4.

Cole MG, Fenton FR, Engelsmann F and Mansouri I (1991) Effectiveness of geriatric psychiatry consultation in an acute care hospital: a randomised clinical trial. *Journal of the American Geriatrics Society* **39**, 118–8.

Cooper AF and Schapira K (1973) Case report: depression, catatonic stupor, and EEG changes in hyperparathyroidism. *Psychological Medicine* **3**, 509–13.

Cooper B (1987) Psychiatric disorders among elderly patients admitted to hospital medical wards. *Journal of the Royal Society of Medicine* **80**, 13–16.

Cushing H (1932) The basophil adenomas of the pituitary body and their clinical manifestations. *Bulletin of the Johns Hopkins Hospital* **50**, 137–95.

Dooneief G, Mirabello E, Bell K et al. (1992) An estimate of the incidence of depression in Parkinson's disease. *Archives of Neurology* **49**, 305–7.

Drinka PJ and Voeks SK (1988) Relationship of depression to hypothyroidism in geriatric patients. *Journal of the American Geriatrics Society* **36**, 284.

Eastwood MR and Corbin SL (1986) The relationship between physical illness and depression in old age. In Murphy E (ed.) *Affective Disorders in the Elderly*. London, Churchill Livingstone.

Eastwood MR, Rifat SL, Nobbs H et al. (1989) Mood disorder following cerebrovascular accident. *British Journal of Psychiatry* **154**, 195–200.

Feldman E, Mayou R, Hawton K et al. (1987) Psychiatric disorder in medical in-patients. *Quarterly Journal of Medicine* **63**, 405–12.

Finch EJL, Ramsay RL, Wright P et al. (1991) Maladies psychiatriques et leurs suites parmi des vieillards hospitalisés d'urgence pour soins medicaux: étude de contrôle à long terme. *Psychologie Medicale* **23**, 735–40.

Fogel BS and Kroessler D (1987) Treating late-life depression on a medical-psychiatric unit. *Hospital and Community Psychiatry* **38**, 829–31.

Folks DG and Ford CV (1985) Psychiatric disorders in geriatric medical/surgical patients. *Southern Medical Journal* **78**, 239–41.

Folstein MF, Maiberger R, McHugh P (1977) Mood disorder as a specific complication of stroke. *Jounal of Neurology, Neurosurgery and Psychiatry* **40** 1018–20.

Fras I, Litin EM and Bartholomew LG (1968) Mental symptoms as an aid in the early diagnosis of carcinoma of the pancreas. *Gastroenterology* **55**, 191–8.

Gaspar D and Samarasinghe LA (1982) ECT in psychogeriatric practice—a study of risk factors, indications and outcome. *Comprehensive Psychiatry* **23**, 17–5.

Gerring JP and Shields HM (1982) The identification and management of patients with a high risk for cardiac arrhythmias during modified ECT. *Journal of Clinical Psychiatry* **43**, 140–3.

Grober SE, Gordon WA, Sliwinski MJ et al. (1991) Utility of the dexamethasone suppression test in the diagnosis of post-stroke depression. *Archives of Physical Medicine and Rehabilitation* **72**, 1076–9.

Gurland BJ, Golden RR, Teresi JA and Challop J (1984) The SHORT-CARE: an efficient instrument for the assessment of depression, dementia and disability. *Journal of Gerontology* **39**, 166–9.

Gurland BJ, Wilder DE, Bolden R et al. (1988) The relationship between depression and disability in the elderly—data from the Comprehensive Assessment and Referral Evaluation (CARE). In Wattis JP and Hindmarsh I (eds) *Psychological Assessment of the Elderly*. Edinburgh, Churchill Livingstone.

Harper RG, Kotik-Harper D and Kirby H (1990) Psychometric assessment of depression in an elderly general medical population. *Journal of Nervous and Mental Disorders* **178**, 113–19.

Harris RE, Mion LC, Patterson MB and Frengley JD (1988) Severe illness in older patients: the association between depressive disorders and functional dependency during the recovery phase. *Journal of the American Geriatrics Society* **36**, 890–6.

House A, Dennis M, Hawton K and Warlow C (1989) Methods of identifying mood disorders in stroke patients: experience in the Oxfordshire Community Stroke Project. *Age and Ageing* **18**, 371–9.

House A, Dennis M, Mogridge L et al. (1991) Mood disorders in the year after first stroke. *British Journal of Psychiatry* **158**, 83–92.

Huber SJ, Paulson GW and Shuttleworth EC (1988) Depression in Parkinson's disease. *Neuropsychiatry, Neuropsychology and Behavioural Neurology* **1**, 47–51.

Johnston M, Wakeling A, Graham N et al. (1987) Cognitive impairment, emotional disorder and length of stay of elderly patients in a district general hospital. *British Journal of Medical Psychology* **60**, 133–9.

Katz IR, Simpson GM, Curlik SM et al. (1990) Pharmacologic treatment of major depression for elderly patients in residential care settings. *Journal of Clinical Psychiatry* **51**, 41–7.

Kitchell MA, Barnes RF, Veith RC et al. (1982) Screening for depression in hospitalised geriatric medical patients. *Journal of the American Geriatrics Society* **30**, 174–7.

Koenig HG, Goli V, Shelp F et al. (1989a) Antidepressant use in elderly medical inpatients: lessons from an attempted clinical trial. *Journal of General and Internal Medicine* **4**, 498–505.

Koenig HG, Meador KG, Cohen HJ et al. (1988a) Depression in elderly hospitalized patients with medical illness. *Archives of Internal Medicine* **148**, 1929–36.

Koenig HG, Meador KG, Cohen HJ et al. (1988b) Detection and treatment of major depression in older medically ill hospitalized patients. *International Journal of Psychiatry in Medicine* **18**, 17–31.

Koenig HG, Meador KG, Cohen HJ et al. (1988c) Self-rated depression scales and screening for major depression in the older hospitalized patient with medical illness. *Journal of the American Geriatrics Society* **36**, 699–706.

Koenig HG, Meador KG, Shelp F et al. (1991) Major depressive disorder in hospitalised medically ill patients: an examination of young and elderly male veterans. *Journal of the American Geriatrics Society* **39**, 881–90.

Koenig HG, Shelp F, Veeraindar G et al. (1989b) Survival and health care utilisation in elderly medical inpatients with major depression. *Journal of the American Geriatrics Society* **37**, 599–606.

Koenig HG and Studenski S (1988) Post-stroke depression in the elderly. *Journal of General and Internal Medicine* **3**, 508–17.

Kua EH (1987) Psychiatric referrals of elderly patients in a general hospital. *Annals of the Academy of Medicine* **16**, 115–17.

Kushnir SL (1986) Lithium-antidepressant combinations in the treatment of depressed, physically ill eriatric patients. *American Journal of Psychiatry* **143**, 378–9.

Lazaro L, de Pablo J, Nieto E et al. (1991) Morbididad psiquiatrica en ancianos ingresados en un hospital general. Estudio prevalencia-dia. *Medical Clinics (Barcelona)* **97**, 206–10.

Lipsey JR, Robinson RG, Pearlson GD et al. (1984) Nortriptyline treatment of post-stroke depression: a double-blind study. *Lancet* **i**, 297–300.

Lishman WA (1987) *Organic Psychiatry* (2nd edn). Oxford, Blackwell Scientific.

Loo H, Cuche H and Benkelfat C (1985) Electroconvulsive therapy during anticoagulant therapy. *Convulsive Therapy* **1**, 258–62.

Mainprize E and Rodin G (1987) Geriatric referrals to a psychiatric consultation-liaison service. *Canadian Journal of Psychiatry* **32**, 5–9.

Marsden CD and Harrison MJG (1972) Outcome of investigation of patents with pre-senile dementia. *British Medical Journal* **2**, 249–53.

Mayeux R, Stern Y, Rosen J et al. (1981) Depression intellectual impairment and Parkinson disease. *Neurology* **31**, 645–50.

Mayeux R, Stern Y, Williams JBW et al. (1986) Clinical and biochemical features of depression in Parkinson's disease. *American Journal of Psychiatry* **143**, 756–9.

Mayou R and Hawton K (1986) Psychiatric morbidity in the general hospital. *British Journal of Psychiatry* **149**, 172–90.

Millar HR (1981) Psychiatric morbidity in eldery surgical patients. *British Journal of Psychiatry* **138**, 17–20.

Mindham RHS (1970) Psychiatric symptoms in Parkinsonism. *Journal of Neurology, Neurosurgery and Psychiatry* **33**, 188–91.

Montgomery SA (1990) Depression in the elderly: pharmacokinetics of antidepressants and death from overdose. *International Clinical Psychopharmacology* Suppl. 3, 67–76.

Murphy E (1983) The prognosis of depression in old age. *British Journal of Psychiatry* **142**, 111–19.

Murphy E, Smith R, Lindesay J et al. (1988) Increased mortality in late life depression. *British Journal of Psychiatry* **152**, 347–53.

O'Riordan TG, Hayes JP, Shelley R et al. (1989) The prevalence of depression in an acute geriatric medical assessment unit. *International Journal of Geriatric Psychiatry* **4**, 17–21.

Parkes CM, Benjamin B and Fitzgerald RG (1969) Broken heart: a statistical study of increased mortality among widowers. *British Medical Journal* **1**, 740.

Pauser H, Bergstrom B and Walinder J (1987) Evaluation of 294 psychiatric consultations involving in-patients above 70 years of age in somatic departments in a university hospital. *Acta Psychiatrica Scandinavica* **76**, 152–7.

Peterson P (1968) Psychiatric disorders in primary hyperparathyroidism. **28**, 1491–5.

Ramsay R, Wright P, Katz A et al. (1991) Psychiatric morbidity and bed-occupancy in geriatric in-patients. *International Journal of Geriatric Psychiatry* **6**, 861–6.

Rapp SR and Davis KM (1989) Geriatric depression: physicians' knowledge, perceptions, and diagnostic practices. *Gerontologist* **29**, 252–7.

Rapp SR, Parisi SA and Wallace CE (1991) Comorbid psychiatric disorders in elderly medical patients: a 1-year prospective study. *Journal of the American Geriatrics Society* **39**, 124–31.

Rapp SR, Parisi SA, Walsh DA et al. (1988a) Detecting depression in elderly medical inpatients. *Journal of Consulting and Clinical Psychology* 56, 509–13.

Rapp SR, Parisi SA and Walsh DA (1988b) Psychological dysfunction and physical health among elderly medical inpatients. *Journal of Consulting and Clinical Psychology* 56, 851–5.

Reding MJ, Orto LA, Winter SW et al. (1986) Antidepressant therapy after stroke: a double-blind trial. *Archives of Neurology* 43, 763–5.

Robins AH (1976) Depression in patient with parkinsonism. *British Journal of Psychiatry* 128, 141–5.

Robinson RG and Price TR (1982) Post-stroke depressive disorders: a follow-up study of 103 patients. *Stroke* 13, 635–41.

Robinson RG and Szetela B (1981) Mood change following left hemispheric brain injury. *Annals of Neurology* 9, 447–53.

Rodin G and Voshart K (1986) Depression in the medically ill: an overview. *American Journal of Psychiatry* 143, 696–705.

Schifano F, Garbin A, Renesto V et al. (1990) A double-blind comparison of mianserin and maprotiline in depressed medically ill elderly people. *Acta Psychiatrica Scandinavica* 81, 289–94.

Schliefer SJ, Keller SE, Siris SG et al. (1985) Depression and immunity. *Archives of General Psychiatry* 42, 129–33.

Schubert DSP, Taylor C, Lee S et al. (1992) Physical consequences of depession in the stroke patient. *General Hospital Psychiatry* 14, 69–76.

Shah A, Phongsathorn V, Bielawska C and Katona CLE (1992) Prevalence of psychiatric morbidity in patients in continuing geriatric care. *International Journal of Geriatric Psychiatry* 7, 517–25.

Shamash K, O'Connell K, Lowy M and Katona CLE (1992) Psychiatric morbidity and outcome in elderly patients undergoing emergency hip surgery. *International Journal of Geriatric Psychiatry* 7, 505–9.

Spitzer RL and Endicott J (1978) Research Diagnostic Criteria for a Selected Group of Functional Disorders (3rd edn). New York, New York State Psychiatric Institute.

Starkstein SE and Robinson RG (1989) Affective disorders and cerebral vascular disease. *British Journal of Psychiatry* 154, 70–182.

Stern RA and Bachman DL (1991) Depressive symptoms following stroke. *American Journal of Psychiatry* 148, 351–6.

Stewart JT (1991) Diagnosing and treati depression in the hospitalised elderly. *Geriatrics* 46, 64–72.

Tappy L, Randin JP, Schwed P et al. (1987) Prevalence of thyroid disorders in psychogeriatric inpatients: a possible relationship of hypothyroidism with neurotic depression but not with dementia. *Journal of the American Geriatrics Society* 35, 526–31.

Wade DT, Legh-Smith J and Hewer RA (1987) Depressed mood after stroke: a community study of its frequency. *British Journal of Psychiatry* 151, 200–5.

Ward L, Stern GM, Pratt RT and McKenna P (198) Electroconvulsive therapy in Parkinsonian patients with the 'on–off' syndrome. *Journal of Neural Transmission* 49, 133–5.

Weizman A, Eldar M, Shoenfeld Y et al. (1979) Hypercalcaemia-induced psychopathology in malignant disease. *British Journal of Psychiatry* 135, 363–6.

Whitlock FA (1978) Suicide, cancer and depression. *British Journal of Psychiatry* 132, 269–74.

Wing JK, Cooper JE and Sartorius N (1974) *The Measurement and Classification of Psychiatric Symptoms*. London, Cambridge University Press.

6 Suicide and Attempted Suicide in Old Age

THE EPIDEMIOLOGY OF SUICIDE IN OLD AGE

It is widely believed that successful suicide is rare in old age. An American study by McIntosh (1985) found that only 29% of the population were aware of the fact that suicide rates are higher among the old than the young, although this is overwhelmingly the case in most countries. In England and Wales, for example, about 30% of suicides occur in subjects aged 65 and over, who represent only 15% of the population (McClure 1984). Stenback (1980) describes a variety of patterns of age-related suicide rate. In males, the three commonest patterns are as follows: steady increases into extreme old age (Austria, Hungary, USA); a peak in the sixth decade with subsequent decline (Canada, Norway, Poland); a similar peak in the sixth decade with a subsequent fall followed by a second peak at age 75 and over (Denmark, Sweden, Switzerland). Patterns for female suicide are similar except that in a number of countries (including Greece and Japan) suicide rates are high in the third and fourth decade and descend to a trough before resuming a progressive upward trend in late-middle and old age.

An analysis of more recent age-related suicide statistics by Pritchard (1992) has confirmed that suicide rates in old age were higher than in the rest of the population in 19 of the 20 countries whose statistics he analysed. He also found a consistent trend for the relative rate of suicide in old age to increase steadily between 1974 and 1987. During this period, male suicide rate in the USA increased by 13% overall but by 35% in those aged 75 and over. The corresponding figures for women were a 20% fall in suicide rates across all ages but a 3% increase in suicide in the elderly.

The epidemiology of suicide in the elderly in the UK across the twentieth century has been comprehensively reviewed by Lindesay (1991) and is summarised in Figure 6.1, which is taken from his paper. In contrast to the more recent international trends reported by Pritchard (1992), suicide rates in the elderly dropped dramatically in the 1960s. The suicide rate in men aged 65 and over was 350 per million in 1961; this was more than seven times the rate in the 15–24 age group. By 1974 this ratio had fallen to about 3:1. This dramatic fall coincided with the

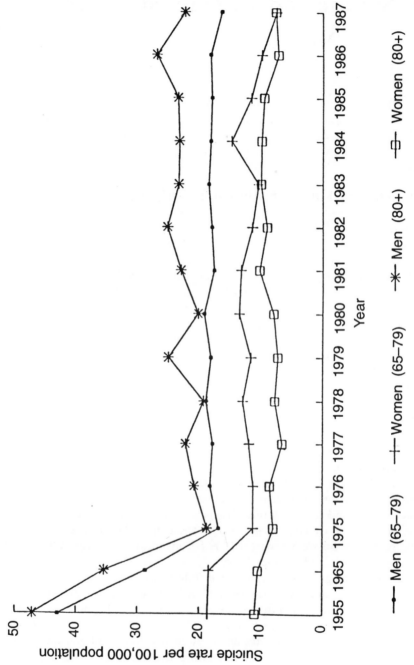

Figure 6.1 Suicide rates in the elderly (65 y+) (England and Wales). From Lindesay (1991), with permission.

introduction of natural gas to replace coal gas for domestic supply, the latter being the favourite method of suicide in the elderly until the 1960s. In more recent years, UK suicide rates have been about 10 per 100,000 for women aged 65 and over with no clear change in rate between the young-old and old-old. In men the rates are approximately double this and slightly higher for those aged 80 and over than those aged 65 to 79.

Lindesay (1991) points out that, apart from the coal gas story, there have been other marked changes in method of suicide in the UK in recent years. Suicide by self-poisoning has decreased steadily due primarily to a fall in rate of barbiturate poisoning. Within self-poisoning deaths, the majority are now due to analgesics and benzodiazepines (Nowers and Irish 1988). In elderly men there has been a marked increase (from 0.4 per 100,000 in 1965 to nearly 2 per 100,000 in 1987) in suicide by car exhaust. De Leo and Ormskerk (1991) have reviewed the question of method of suicide in the elderly in an international context. In general men are more likely to use violent means than women. In the USA the overwhelming majority of elderly men who kill themselves do so by violent means, particularly shooting. Conwell et al. (1990), in a retrospective case-note survey of 246 USA suicides aged 50 and over, found that 64% used violent means. Both in men and women the proportion using such means increased significantly with increasing age. In most other western countries, 85% of suicides are by self-poisoning, jumping, hanging and car exhaust inhalation.

The relationship between age and suicide may, like that linking age and depression (see Chapter 4), reflect cohort effects as well as those directly attributable to age itself. Period effects such as wars, changes in the prescribing of hypnotic drugs and detoxification of domestic gas supplies may further confound the issue. Lindesay (1991) considers that period effects may be particularly important in the elderly, who are less likely than their younger counterparts to find new means of suicide following the removal of a popular method. USA figures (analysed by Blazer et al. 1986) suggest relatively consistent suicide rates within birth cohorts but a steady decline in suicide rate between those born in 1892 and those born in 1922. Significant age-related increases in suicide rate after the age of 75 were, however, apparent in all the cohorts. The British study by Murphy et al. (1986) did not, however, find evidence of either consistently increased risk of suicide across birth cohorts or a consistent pattern of progressive increase in suicide rates within given age groups across cohorts.

Gender may be an important confounding variable as well as having a direct effect on suicide rates. Woodbury et al. (1988) have noted that the relationship between age and suicide remained linear in men into extreme old age, whereas in women suicide risk peaked in the years surrounding the menopause with a subsequent decline.

Despite the complexity of interactions between these age, period, cohort and gender effects, it is clear that there is no room for complacency in terms either of the high absolute rate of suicide in old age or the tendency for the proportion of elderly suicides to increase.

PSYCHIATRIC ILLNESS AND SUICIDE IN OLD AGE

Several studies have used the technique of 'psychiatric autopsy' to make retrospective diagnoses on the basis of detailed interviews with nearest relatives supplemented by examination of primary care and hospital case notes in consecutive series of suicide victims. This approach, which requires clear evidence of a range of clinical features in order to permit a psychiatric diagnosis, is important in avoiding the circular argument of regarding the suicidal act itself as evidence of psychiatric illness or more specifically of depression. Early studies both in the USA (Dorpat and Ripley 1960, Robins et al. 1960) and in the UK (Barraclough et al.1974), and more recent studies in the USA (Rich et al. 1986), Australia (Chynoweth et al. 1980) and Hungary (Arato et al. 1988) have concluded that the overwhelming majority of suicides (over 90% in most studies) are associated with specific psychiatric illness. The most frequent diagnosis, occurring in approximately 50% of the total, is depression.

The majority of these studies have not examined an elderly subsample separately. A notable exception to this is the work of Barraclough (1971), who carried out a more detailed assessment of the 30 subjects from the series of 100 reported by Barraclough et al. (1974) who were aged 65 and over. Twenty-six (87%) had depressive illnesses, though in seven the depression was associated with terminal physical illness, alcoholism or acute confusional state. None had dementia. Within the depressed suicides a number of specific symptoms were common, notably insomnia (90%), weight loss (75%) and hypochondriasis (50%). Depression did not appear to be particularly severe in terms of psychotic features, hypochondriasis, marked motor abnormalities or profoundly depressed mood. Half had been ill for six months or less and the same proportion had consulted their GPs within the week before their deaths. As many as 90% had consulted their GPs within the three months prior to their death but hardly any were regarded as either potentially violent or actively suicidal by either their relatives or their doctors. As few as six (20%) were prescribed antidepressants and only three (10%) were receiving them in therapeutically adequate doses.

Several more recent studies have provided support for these findings, in particular that a link between depression and suicide is particularly close in old age and that most elderly suicide victims have had recent contact with their doctors, representing a potential chance for intervention.

Conwell et al. (1991) found that within 18 suicides aged 50 years and over, unipolar major depression was diagnosed in 12 (67%) with a further 3 (13%) having dysthymic disorder. Carlson et al. (1991) carried out a systematic comparison in age group bands between the cohorts of male suicides studied by Robins et al. (1960) and Rich et al. (1986). The findings within the elderly cohorts (age 61 and over) are somewhat surprising in that, although affective disorder was present in 53% in the earlier cohort, that figure had fallen to 18.5% in the later one. It should be noted, however, that the majority of elderly subjects in the later study received 'other' (unspecified) diagnoses which, the authors state, represented people with organic brain syndromes and those on whom insufficient data was available to make a diagnosis. The greater difficulty of making retrospective diagnoses in elderly suicides may reflect the fact that elderly people with severe psychiatric illness who are at high risk of suicide may be less likely than their younger counterparts to be referred for specialist psychiatric help. In keeping with this, Conwell et al. (1990) found that only 53 out of 246 completed suicides in people aged over 50 had documented psychiatric illness, though of these nearly half had affective disorders. Within the sample, increasing age was associated with decreasing likelihood of psychiatric contact, contact rate being 49% in the 50–55 age range and only 25% in those aged 74 and over.

As far as GP contact is concerned, Mellick et al. (1992) reported that 77% of their small series of 18 subjects had contacted their GPs within the month prior to their death. Similarly, Conwell et al. (1991) noted that 7 of the 18 subjects they studied had seen their GP during their last week of life.

The clear relationship between suicide and psychiatric illness indicates that identified psychiatric patients (especially those with a diagnosis of depression) may be at particularly high risk. Elderly depressed patients have a risk of suicide about four times as great as their younger counterparts (Tobias et al. 1992). Modestin (1989) examined the age distribution of a consecutive series of psychiatric inpatient suicides and found that 15% were aged 60 years or more. This proportion was no greater than in non-suicide admissions. Formal comparisons between elderly and younger suicides and between the elderly suicide group and elderly non-suicide admissions revealed few differences. Sixty-four per cent of the elderly suicides had an RDC (Spitzer and Endicott 1978) diagnosis of depression. Elderly suicides had significantly more frequent previous admissions than elderly controls and were strikingly more likely to have had long index admissions: 45% had been in hospital for more than a year compared with only 10% of controls.

ATTEMPTED SUICIDE IN OLD AGE

Several studies have suggested that clinical characteristics of suicides and attempted suicides are more similar in old age and that attempted suicide in the elderly carries a higher risk of subsequent completed suicide. In a study of attempted suicides in Sheffield over a two-year period, Parkin and Stengel (1965) found that the ratio of suicide attempts to completed suicide was 20:1 in the 20–40 year age group in contrast with 4:1 in the over-60s. Though two-thirds of the elderly suicide attempters in this series were female, more than two-thirds of those who subsequently killed themselves were male. This is in keeping with the findings of Kreitman (1976), who examined a cohort of 822 patients attempting suicide and admitted to the Edinburgh Royal Infirmary. Subjects were divided into 15–34, 35–54 and over-55 age groups; 58% of the elderly subjects were women (a similar proportion to that in younger groups). At three-year follow-up, 8% of the older males and 3% of the older females had successfully committed suicide, both figures being considerably higher than in the younger groups. Older subjects also had an over-representation of chronic physical illness and nearly two-thirds of them had clear-cut depressive illnesses. Organic syndromes were rarer (less than 10%) and compared with younger subjects, elderly suicide attempters showed an under-representation of alcoholism and personality disorder.

The high prevalence of psychiatric illness (particularly depression) in elderly suicide attempters has been confirmed by four more recent studies restricted to the elderly. Their findings are summarised in Table 6.1. The American study by Frierson (1991) reported 61% of subjects to be male in contrast with an excess of women in each of the British studies (Nowers 1990; Pierce 1987; Upadhyaya et al. 1989). A further contrast between the British and American studies is that the overwhelming majority of subjects in each of the recent British reports ingested tablets as their method of deliberate self-harm, whereas Frierson (1991) found that only 43% took overdoses, most of the remainder using violent means (gunshot wounds 34%, wrist cutting 6.3%, stabbing 5.3%). This mirrors the international differences in mode of completed suicide discussed earlier.

Medical ill health appeared to be the single most important precipitant of suicidal behaviour in each of the above series. Peirce (1987) reported such illness to be present in 63%; Nowers (1990) reported a figure of 49% (with chronic physical illness being more frequently found in females); the corresponding figures in Frierson (1991) and Upadhyaya et al. (1989) were 48% and 46% respectively. Subsequent suicide rates (with variable follow-up intervals) ranged between 6% (Nowers 1990) and 3% (Pierce 1987).

These studies strongly support the notion that suicidal behaviour in elderly people is a much more specific marker of high suicide risk than is the case in younger deliberate self-harmers. This is borne out in a study of suicide attempts in elderly psychiatric inpatients by Lyness et al. (1992), in which 25/168 (15%) of subjects made a suicide attempt during their index admission. Eighty per cent of attempters had a major depressive syndrome, though it should be noted that a similar proportion (75%) of the non-attempters had the same diagnosis. Attempted suicide was commoner in those subjects in whom the depression was accompanied by psychotic features or stupor.

Table 6.1 psychiatric diagnoses in attempted suicide

	Depression (%)	Alcoholism (%)	Organic psychoses (%)	Other/ unspecified (%)
Pierce (1987)	93	12	5	—
Upadhyaya et al. (1989)	57	—	2	22
Nowers (1990)	64	11	8	17
Frierson (1991)	64	8	3	31

THE AETIOLOGY OF SUICIDE AND ATTEMPTED SUICIDE IN OLD AGE

We have already seen that psychiatric illness, particularly depression, may be important in the aetiology of suicide and attempted suicide in old age. Vogel and Wolfersdorf (1989) emphasise, however, that the mere demonstration of psychiatric illness in the weeks or months prior to suicide does not necessarily make the psychiatric illness a sufficient explanation in itself. In a study of 310 psychiatric inpatients, of whom 24 were aged 65 or over, they examined motivation for suicide, as elicited from clinical files, questioning ward staff and personal recollections. Elderly subjects were more likely than their younger counterparts to have committed suicide in the context of family conflict, recent bereavement, subjective and/or objective experience of loneliness and the presence of chronic incurable disease. The authors suggest that high suicide rates in old age reflect the increased loneliness and isolation of older people rather than simply their increased psychiatric morbidity. The question of motivation for suicide has also been examined by Kerkhof et al. (1991), in whose view suicide is best understood as a response to a situation felt to be unbearable. In the elderly, such unbearable states are related most frequently to severe physical suffering, bereavement, the threat of dependency and severely disturbed social relations.

The theme of suicide in old age being related to loss is taken up in several other studies. Barraclough (1971) found that nearly half the elderly suicides he studied were permanently living alone compared with only 20% of the local older population as a whole. Though bereavement was the cause of living alone in about one-third of the subjects Barraclough studied, it is important to note that, as Stenback (1980) points out, the contribution of bereavement to the aetiology of suicide may best be understood through the depression that it all too frequently elicits (see Chapter 4). De Leo and Ormskerk (1991) have reviewed the literature on marital status and suicide in old age. They conclude that being married is associated with a substantially decreased risk of suicide. This is particularly the case in men, in whom divorced, widowed and unmarried subjects have three times the suicide rate of their married counterparts. It must be remembered, however, that marital status and social isolation are closely inter-related. Since social isolation is more frequent and therefore expected in elderly people as a whole, it is perhaps not surprising that, as Whitlock (1973) has observed, 'social and environment circumstances have greater impact on younger suicides than they do on the oldest age groups'. A particular such variable that may be an exception to this rule, however, is moving house. Sainsbury (1973), who has examined the relationship between moving house and suicide in great detail, has concluded that elderly men and middle-aged women are in fact the groups most vulnerable to the increased suicide risk associated with recent house move. In his view this is because adjustment to a new environment is particularly difficult in late life.

It is, of course, likely that the variables discussed above are closely inter-related. House move, for example, is not a randomly occurring event and is particularly likely to occur in the context of major (and often adverse) changes in life circumstances such as increased dependency necessitating a move to residential care. One such change that has already been seen (Chapter 4) to be particularly important in the aetiology of depression in old age is deterioration in physical health. This also appears to be linked to increased suicide risk in old age. In the study by Barraclough (1971), 17 subjects out of 30 had important physical disorders compared with only 9 out of 30 consecutive accidental deaths matched for age and sex. Richardson et al. (1989) have emphasised the wide range of loss events (physical, occupational, economic, social and cognitive) associated with ageing and suggest that the desire to die may be a reflection not just of one particular loss but of the accumulation of many.

Biological variables may also be important in the aetiology of suicide in old age. Lindesay (1991) has raised the possibility that, since suicidal acts are associated with reductions in serotonergic functioning and that similar reductions occur with aging, this might explain the vulnerability of some elderly individuals to suicide. This argument is reviewed in greater detail by Rifai et al. (1992), who conclude that there is little evidence as yet within studies of post-mortem suicide brain to implicate age as a significant factor but that this would be a fruitful area for further research. A notable study by Jones et al. (1990) has compared cerebrospinal fluid concentrations of major metabolites of noradrenaline (5HIAA) and dopamine (HVA) in a series of 12 elderly depressed patients who attempted suicide as well as 9 age-matched depressed patients without a history of suicide attempt and 7 normal elderly controls. The two depressed groups were similar in severity of depression, degree of expressed hostility and history of recent life events, but CSF levels of both metabolites were significantly lower in the attempted suicide group. Despite the small numbers in the study, it provides at least some evidence that the relative contribution of biological factors to suicidal behaviour in old age may be considerable.

STRATEGIES FOR MANAGING ATTEMPTED SUICIDE AND REDUCING SUICIDE RISK IN OLD AGE

The main contribution individual practitioners (in primary care or psychiatry) can make to the prevention of suicide is to acquire the clinical skills to recognise individual patients at high risk and to manage them appropriately. A number of clinical features (summarised in Table 6.2) should alert practitioners to careful consideration of the possibility of suicide in their elderly patients. Most important among such indicators is, of course, any expressed wish to die or any act of deliberate self-harm. As we have seen, elderly people who harm themselves have a clinical profile much more like that of completed suicides than is the case for younger patients; the likelihood that an elderly person who commits an act of self-harm will subsequently end his or her life is correspondingly higher. A number of specific clinical features and behaviours may also be useful as indicators

Table 6.2   Risk factors for suicide in old age

Demographic/general
  Male
  Living alone
  Not married
  Socially isolated
  Recent bereavement
  Recent house move

Individual/clinical
  Expresses wish to harm self
  Anhedonia
  Prominent depressive cognition (guilt, helplessness, hopelessness)
  Personal affairs put in order (e.g. new will)
  Persistent complaints of insomnia
  Persistent physical symptoms without organic basis
  Weight loss
  Chronic physical ill health

of high suicide risk. In particular expressed feelings of helplessness, hopelessness or guilt and the development of anhedonia (the loss of the capacity to enjoy) should be taken very seriously. Elderly patients who without clear reason put their financial affairs in order, give away their possessions, and/or start neglecting themselves may also be harbouring suicidal thoughts.

Practitioners are often concerned that their questions about suicidal ideation may actually put the suicidal ideas into their patients heads; this is very unlikely to be the case. Indeed though elderly people often feel particularly guilty about such thoughts, careful and sympathetic questioning may allow them to unburden themselves. This may prove the beginning of a useful therapeutic intervention.

The demographic characteristics and recent life experiences of elderly patients may themselves provide some clue as to degree of suicide risk. Those living alone, particularly as a result of recent bereavement, and those who have recently moved house may appropriately give cause for specific concern. Patients who have recently experienced major deterioration in their physical health may also be at high risk as may those who, in the absence of objective evidence of poor physical health, continue to complain bitterly of aches, pains and poor sleep. Patients seldom become querulous and irritating to their doctors for no reason, and suicide risk should be considered particularly in such patients.

The relationship between psychiatric illness (particularly depression) and suicide has been described in some detail above. From the point of view of detecting patients at risk of suicides, it is important for GPs and hospital practitioners alike to have a high index of suspicion for depression in their elderly patients. The use of screening instruments for depression, such as the Geriatric Depression Scale (Yesavage et al. 1983; see also Chapter 2) may be particularly useful in this context.

It is also important for non-psychiatrists involved in the care of elderly patients to be very critical of their patients' apparently rational wish to die. Simon (1989) has highlighted the importance of 'silent suicide' in the elderly. Such patients try to kill themselves by non-violent means through self-starvation or non-compliance with treatment. They usually have underlying and undiagnosed depressive illnesses and it is of great importance to distinguish such patients from those with true terminal illness. Relatives and clinicians alike may fall into the trap of assuming that nothing can be done or that the patient is better left alone. From a legal point of view, an elderly patient's competence to refuse treatment must not be assumed uncritically in the absence of terminal physical disease and where the possibility of underlying and treatable depression has not been explored. In a recent editorial on this subject, Conwell and Caine (1991) conclude that 'suicide in the absence of treatable affective illness is uncommon among the old . . . to the extent that clinical depressive illness precludes rational decision making, the proportion of rational self-inflicted deaths does not increase with age'. As far as psychiatrists are concerned, it is clear that the patients they see who are most at risk are those with depressive illnesses, though such depressions need neither be particularly severe or chronic. Osgood (1987) has emphasised that elderly patients who abuse alcohol, particularly those in whom such abuse is of late onset and in response to loss and social isolation, may also be at very high risk of suicide.

Once individual patients at high risk have been recognised, there are a number of principles of treatment that should be considered. The first is the avoidance of therapeutic nihilism; most such patients have treatable psychiatric illnesses and degrees of loss and social isolation which are amenable to environmental and psychotherapeutic intervention. Tobias et al. (1992) have suggested that a useful first step in the management of elderly patients at high suicide risk is the making of a verbal or written 'contract' against suicide. In their view, patients usually abide by such a promise and in particular by an agreement to contact the physician again should suicidal wishes become more pressing. Hospitalisation is often helpful at least until treatment of the underlying psychiatric illness is established. In the series of attempted suicides reviewed by Pierce (1987),nearly half the patients were admitted to inpatient psychiatric care, a very much higher proportion than would be expected in a younger population. The objective measurement of suicide risk may be helpful in the decision whether or not to hospitalise. Pierce (1987) found that scores on the suicidal intent scale of Beck et al. (1974) were significantly higher in patients admitted to hospital than in those not admitted and, more importantly, were very much higher in those who later committed suicide. The use of such a scale in guiding management decisions in elderly patients following deliberate self-harm may, therefore, be very useful and this approach certainly deserves further evaluation.

Appropriate treatment of underlying depression should follow the same principles as are outlined in Chapter 7. There is some evidence in younger patients that antidepressants acting primarily on the serotonergic system may be particularly effective in reducing suicidal ideation (Muijen et al. 1988). These drugs are also relatively safe in overdose and therefore may represent the best drugs of first choice for elderly patients with suicidal ideation.

Strategies for the primary prevention of suicide in old age need a political as well as a clinical dimension. If both depression and suicide are to be understood at least in part in terms of the multiple losses experienced in old age, it is clear that enabling a high proportion of old people to have a good quality old age is likely to be the most effective way of reducing their suicide rate. In view of the evidence that elderly people contemplating suicide are less able than their younger counterparts to change from established methods of suicide it is likely that changes in prescribing habits and the availability of firearms may also be helpful. Decreases in the use of benzodiazepines for more than very short periods should make such drugs less available to older patients contemplating suicide, as may a switch towards the use of less toxic antidepressant drugs (Lindesay 1991). Changes in car exhaust systems leading to much lower emissions of carbon monoxide may also be useful. Lindesay (1991) has also pointed out that the widespread practice of prescribing tricyclic antidepressants at sub-therapeutic doses to elderly depressed patients may provide them for long periods with the means to kill themselves without any associated likelihood of alleviating their depression. The same applies to the still frequent practice of prescribing sedative tricyclic anti-depressants in low doses to elderly patients for purely hypnotic purposes. Any elderly patient newly requesting hypnotics should be screened for depression and in particular for suicidal ideation. Primary sleep disturbance in old age seldom warrants drug treatment, though depression associated with sleep disturbance may be appropriately and rewardingly treated with antidepressant drugs even where such drugs do not have a direct sedating effect.

REFERENCES

Arato M, Demeter Z, Rihmer Z and Somogyi E (1988) Retrospective psychiatric assessment of 200 suicides in Budapest. *Acta Psychiatrica Scandinavica* **77**, 454–6.

Barraclough BM (1971) Suicide in the elderly. In Kay DWK and Walk A (eds) *Recent Developments in Psychogeriatrics*, pp. 87–97. Ashford, Headley Bros.

Barraclough M, Bunch J, Nelson B et al. (1974) One hundred cases of suicide—clinical aspects. *British Journal of Psychiatry* **125**, 355–73.

Beck AT, Schuyler D and Herman J (1974) Development of suicide intent scales. In Beck AT, Resnick L and Lettieri BBG (eds) *Prediction of Suicide*. Maryland, Charles Press.

Blazer DG, Bachar JR and Manton KG (1986) Suicide in late life: review and commentary. *Journal of the American Geriatrics Society* **34**, 519–25.

Carlson GA, Rich CL, Grayson P and Fowler RC (1991) Secular trends in the psychiatric diagnoses of suicide victims. *Journal of Affective Disorders* **21**, 127–32.

Chynoweth R, Tonge JI and Armstrong J (1980) Suicide in Brisbane: a retrospective psychological study. *Australia and New Zealand Journal of Psychiatry* **14**, 37–45.

Conwell Y and Caine ED (1991) Rational suicide and the right to die: reality and myth. *New England Journal of Medicine* **325**, 1100–3.

Conwell Y, Olsen K, Caine ED and Flannery C (1991) Suicide in later life: psychological autopsy findings. *International Psychogeriatrics* **3**, 59–66.

Conwell Y, Rotenberg M and Caine ED (1990) Completed suicide at age 50 and over. *Journal of the American Geriatrics Society* **38**, 640–4.

De Leo D and Ormskerk SCR (1991) Suicide in the elderly: general characteristics. *Crisis* **12**, 3–17.

Dorpat TL and Ripley HS (1960) A study of suicide in the Seattle area. *Comprehensive Psychiatry* **1**, 349–59.

Frierson RL (1991) Suicide attempts by the old and the very old. *Archives of Internal Medicine* **151**, 141–4.

Jones JS, Stanley B, Mann JJ et al. (1990) CSF 5-HIAA and HVA concentrations in elderly depressed patients who attempted suicide. *American Journal of Psychiatry* **147**, 1225–7.

Kerkhof AJFM, Visser AP, Diekstra RFW and Hirschhorn PM (1991) The prevention of suicide among older people in The Netherlands: interventions in community health care. *Crisis* **12**, 59–72.

Kreitman N (1976) Age and parasuicide. *Psychological Medicine* **6**, 113–21.

Lindesay J (1991) Suicide in the elderly. *International Journal of Geriatric Psychiatry* **6**, 355–61.

Lyness JM, Conwell Y and Nelson JC (1992) Suicide attempts in elderly psychiatric patients. *Journal of the American Psychiatric Association* **40**, 320–4.

McClure GMG (1984) Trends in suicide rate for England and Wales 1975–1980. *British Journal of Psychiatry*, **144**, 119–26.

McIntosh JL (1985) Suicide among the elderly: levels and trends. *American Journal of Orthopsychiatry* **55**, 288–93.

Mellick E, Buckwalter KC and Stolley JM (1992) Suicide among elderly white men: development of a profile. *Journal of Psychosocial Nursing* **30**, 29–34.

Modestin J (1989) Completed suicide in psychogeriatric inpatients. *International Journal of Geriatric Psychiatry* **4**, 209–14.

Muijen M, Roy D, Silverstone T et al. (1988) A comparative clinical trial of fluoxetine, mianserin and placebo with depressed out-patients. *Acta Psychiatrica Scandinavica* **78**, 384–90.

Murphy E, Lindesay J and Grundy E (1986) 60 years of suicide in England and Wales: a cohort study. *Archives of General Psychiatry* **43**, 969–76.

Nowers M (1990) Deliberate self-harm in the elderly. MPhil thesis, University of London.

Nowers M and Irish M (1988) Trends in the reported rates of suicide by self-poisoning in the elderly. *Journal of the Royal College of General Practitioners* **38**, 67–9.

Osgood NJ (1987) The alcohol–suicide connection in late life. *Postgraduate Medicine* **81**, 379–84.

Parkin D and Stengel E (1965) Incidence of suicide attempts in an urban community. *British Medical Journal* **ii**, 133–8.

Pierce D (1987) Deliberate self-harm in the elderly. *International Journal of Geriatric Psychiatry* **2**, 105–10.

Pritchard C (1992) Changes in elderly suicides in the USA and the developed world 1974–87: comparison with current homicide. *International Journal of Geriatric Psychiatry* **7**, 125–34.

Rich CL, Young D and Fowler RC (1986) San Diego suicide study: 1. Young vs old subjects. *Archives of General Psychiatry* **43**, 577–82.

Richardson R, Lowenstein S and Weissberg M (1989) Coping with the suicidal elderly: a physician's guide. *Geriatrics* **44**, 43–51.

Rifai AH, Reynolds CF and Mann JJ (1992) Biology of elderly suicide. *Suicide and Life-Threatening Behaviour* **22**, 48–61.

Robins E, Murphy GE, Wilkinson RH et al. (1960) Some clinical considerations in the prevention of suicide based on a study of 134 successful suicides. *American Journal of Public Health* **49**, 888–98.

Sainsbury P (1973) Suicide: opinions and facts. *Proceedings of the Royal Society of Medicine* **66**, 579–87.

Simon RI (1989) Silent suicide in the elderly. *Bulletin of the American Academy of Psychiatry and Law* **17**, 83–95.

Spitzer RL and Endicott J (1978) *Research Diagnostic Criteria for a Selected Group of Functional Disorders* (3rd edn) New York, New York State Psychiatric Institute.

Stenback A (1980) Depression and suicidal behaviour in old age. In Birren JE and Slone RB (Ed) *Handbook of Mental Health and Aging*. Englewood Cliffs, NJ, Prentice-Hall.

Tobias CR, Pary R and Lippmann S (1992) Preventing suicide in older people. *American Family Physician* **45**, 1707–13.

Upadhyaya AK, Warburton H and Jenkins JC (1989) Psychiatric correlates of non-fatal deliberate self-harm in the elderly: a pilot study. *Journal of Clinical and Experimental Gerontology* **11**, 131–143.

Vogel R and Wolfersdorf M (1989) Suicide and mental illness in the elderly. *Psychopathology* **22**, 202–7.

Whitlock FA (1973) Suicide in England and Wales 1959–63. Part 1. The county boroughs. *Psychological Medicine* **3**, 350–65.

Woodbury MA, Manton KG and Blazer D (1988) Trends in US mortality rates 1968 to 1982: race and sex differences in age, period and cohort components. *International Journal of Epidemiology* **17**, 356–62.

Yesavage JA, Brink TL, Rose TL and Lum 0 (1983) Development and validation of a geriatric depression screening scale: a preliminary report. *Journal of Psychiatric Research* **17**, 37–49.

7 The Management of Depression in Old Age

In this chapter, the use of antidepressant drugs, electroconvulsive therapy (ECT) and psychological treatments will be considered. In general, of course, the same principles of management apply as for younger depressed patients. Above all, in elderly as in younger patients it is unlikely that a single treatment modality will be adequate. Management must be holistic, and appropriate medical and social interventions to reduce disability and isolation are likely to contribute as much to the resolution of depression in old age as any more specific treatment for depression. The role of the multidisciplinary team (at both primary care and hospital levels) is crucial not only to ensure that a holistic view to patient care prevails but also for service coordination. In particular, Blanchard et al. (1994) have shown that a nurse can be an effective coordinator of care delivery for elderly depressed patients.

There are, however, a number of particular problems in treating the depressions of old age, associated mainly with age-related changes in drug handling and in cognitive function, which need to be considered when planning the treatment of individual patients.

TRICYCLIC ANTIDEPRESSANTS AND MONOAMINE-OXIDASE INHIBITORS (MAOIs) AND THEIR LIMITATIONS

The use of tricyclic antidepressants and monoamine-oxidase inhibitors (MAOIs) in elderly patients is often problematic. There is considerable evidence that elderly patients are more likely to suffer antidepressant-related side-effects and to develop more serious adverse consequences as a result. The side-effects of particular relevance in the elderly are summarised in Table 7.1. Perhaps most important is the fact that elderly patients are more vulnerable to falls (Campbell 1991). This is due in large part to orthostatic hypotension, since even in the absence of exposure to antidepressants, baroreceptor reflexes are blunted with increasing age (Woodhouse 1992). The sedative effects of many antidepressants may also increase the risk of falls, the consequences of which are also likely to be more severe because patients with age-related osteoporosis are more vulnerable to suffer fractures as a result of falls. Elderly patients' cognitive function is also more likely

Table 7.1   Side-effects of tricyclic antidepressants
of particular relevance in older patients

Anticholinergic
    Confusion
    Urinary retention
    Precipitation/worsening of glaucoma
    Blurring of vision
Antihistaminic
    Sedation
Antiadrenergic
    Postural hypotension
    Dizziness
    Falls

---

to be impaired by antidepressants with powerful anticholinergic effects (Moskowitz and Burns 1986).

Age-related pharmacokinetic changes also increase the potential of antidepressants to cause side-effects. Since most tricyclics are extensively protein bound, age-related decreases in protein synthesis can increase free plasma drug levels. Reduced creatinine clearance and reduced hepatic blood flow may also contribute to increased blood levels of tricyclics by delaying their excretion. It must, however, be borne in mind that inter-individual variability in blood levels of tricyclics and their active metabolites is considerable in elderly as well as in younger subjects. Thus, in the absence of routinely available plasma level monitoring (and with the exception of nortriptyline for which plasma levels should remain within a 'therapeutic window'), titration to maximum tolerated dose may be as necessary in elderly as in younger subjects, though the average dose required will be smaller.

Despite the need to monitor its levels closely, nortriptyline has been found to be relatively free of the problems associated with other tricyclics in elderly subjects. An open study of nortriptyline in elderly and younger depressed patients (Kanba et al. 1992) found no difference in likelihood of adverse effects between older and younger subjects and no age-related increase in blood level achieved for a given dose. In keeping with this, Miller et al. (1991) found that only 5 out of a series of 45 elderly depressed subjects given nortriptyline in an open trial were unable to tolerate the drug. In general, side-effects decreased as severity of depression fell with treatment. Specifically, no nortriptyline-associated increase in orthostatic hypotension was seen.

DO CONVENTIONAL ANTIDEPRESSANTS WORK IN THE ELDERLY?

Surprisingly few studies have examined the efficacy of these drugs against placebo in patients over the age of 60. The reviews by Gerson et al. (1988) and Rockwell et al. (1988) identified only one placebo-controlled evaluation of amitriptyline (Branconnier et al. 1982), three of imipramine (Gerner et al. 1980; Meredith et al. 1984; Wakelin et al. 1986) and none of desipramine or trimipramine. Single placebo-controlled studies of the MAOIs iproniazid (Shapiro et al. 1960) and phenelzine (Georgotas et al. 1986) have also been performed. Three studies (Georgotas et al. 1987; Katz et al. 1990; Lipsey et al. 1984) have evaluated nortriptyline (which, as discussed above, may be particularly well tolerated by elderly subjects) against placebo in elderly patients. The study by Katz et al. (1990) was performed in a residential care setting and that by Lipsey et al. (1984), which is discussed in Chapter 5, with stroke patients. It is noteworthy that nortriptyline has also recently been found in an open trial to induce significant reductions in HDRS scores in elderly patients with bereavement-related depression, but not to affect the intensity of their grief.

Although all the placebo-controlled studies found the active compound to be superior it must be remembered that most of the elderly patients met with in routine clinical practice would not qualify for such clinical trials. The majority fulfil DSM III or DSM IIIR (American Psychiatric Association 1980, 1987) criteria for dysthymia rather than major depressive episode (Kivela et al. 1988), the latter forming the standard entry criterion for antidepressant trials in elderly as in younger subjects. Equally important, many have one or more medical contra-indications to the use of tricyclic antidepressants (Mullan et al. 1994). A further problem with evaluative studies of antidepressants in the elderly is that the outcome measures, like the inclusion criteria, are geared towards a younger population. As discussed in Chapter 2, rating scales like the Hamilton Depression Rating Scale (HDRS; Hamilton 1960), which have a heavy weighting of somatic items, are likely to be distorted in elderly patients by the coexistence of physical disease. It is thus unlikely that the relationship between change in scale score and true antidepressant response will be the same as in younger patients. Less age-related distortion in results would be seen if global response scales such as the Clinical Global Impression (CGI); scales specifically designed to measure change in elderly depressed subjects like the Geriatric Depression Scale (GDS; Yesavage et al. 1983); or less somatic symptom laden scales like the Montgomery–Asberg Depression Rating Scale (MADRS; Montgomery and Asberg 1979) were used. Evidence for long-term efficacy of tricyclic antidepressants in preventing relapse in elderly patients is relatively lacking (see Chapter 8). It is worth noting at this point, however, that the recent OADIG trial (Old Age Depression Interest Group 1993) found that, compared with placebo, dothiepin reduced relative risk of depressive relapse (over a two-year period) by two and a half times.

At a more practical level, drugs that need to be taken many times a day and at more than one tablet per dose are less likely to be complied with by elderly patients. Age-related increases in vulnerability to other diseases and likelihood of receiving other treatments makes elderly patients more vulnerable to drug–drug and drug–disease interactions. There is some evidence that tricyclic antidepressants may take a surprisingly long time to be effective in elder patients with useful effects sometimes only emerging in the seventh and eighth week of treatment (Georgotas et al. 1989).

In the light of this it is perhaps not surprising that primary care physicians and psychiatrists show considerable reluctance to treat elderly patients with antidepressants. Macdonald (1986) found that although primary care physicians were able to identify most of the depressed elderly patients under their care they hardly ever either initiated treatment themselves or made psychiatric referrals. Similarly, Copeland et al. (1992) found that only 4% of a community sample of elderly depressed patients received treatment.

PROFILE OF THE 'IDEAL ANTIDEPRESSANT' FOR THE ELDERLY

It is, therefore, clear that, theoretically at least, the 'ideal antidepressant' would differ considerably from the tricyclics. In particular, such an ideal drug would show unchanged pharmacokinetics with aging, be free of interactions with other drugs commonly used in the elderly and be safely administered even to frail elderly patients with concomitant physical disease. The ideal drug would also have a simple once daily dosage regime and have proven efficacy both against established comparator drugs and placebo in intention-to-treat (ITT) as well as completer (COMP) analyses, since only the former take drop-out rates into account. Such trials should be of epidemiologically representative samples and use clinically valid measures of antidepressant response. Further requirements for an ideal drug would include good side-effect profile, rapid onset of antidepressant action and demonstrable efficacy in relapse prevention.

STUDIES OF NEWER ANTIDEPRESSANTS IN THE ELDERLY

As well as the novel tricyclic antidepressant lofepramine, four serotonin-specific re-uptake inhibitors (SSRIs; fluvoxamine, fluoxetine, paroxetine and sertraline) and one 'new generation' monoamine-oxidase inhibitor (moclobemide), are currently available for clinical use in the UK and have been evaluated in elderly patients. The remainder of this section will review the controlled trial evidence concerning the efficacy of these newer antidepressants in comparison with established antidepressants and where possible placebo, seeking to discover whether they represent any significant progress towards an ideal antidepressant for elderly patients. The trial results are summarised in Table 7.2.

LOFEPRAMINE

Lofepramine has a conventional tricyclic structure but *in vitro* studies and trials in non-elderly subjects suggest that it is relatively free of anticholinergic side-effects Sjogren 1980). The effects of single doses of lofepramine (70–140 mg) have been compared with 50 mg amitriptyline and placebo in drug-free healthy elderly volunteers. Side-effects of lofepramine and placebo did not differ significantly. Amitriptyline, however, was associated with more frequent subjective side-effects than either lofepramine or placebo. Standing diastolic blood pressure was also reduced in comparison with lofepramine and salivary volume (an objective measure of dry mouth) reduced in comparison with both placebo and lofepramine. Though amitriptyline also impaired performance on choice reaction time, lofepramine was associated with significantly better choice recognition time than placebo (Ghose and Sedman 1987). The same group (Ghose and Spragg 1989) examined the pharmacokinetics of single doses of lofepramine and amitriptyline in healthy drug-free elderly subjects. They found the elimination half-life of lofepramine to be 2.5 hours (compared with 31 hours for amitriptyline), but noted very great inter-individual variation in peak plasma lofepramine concentrations. These studies suggest that lofepramine has unchanged pharmacokinetics compared with younger subjects despite its very extensive (99%) protein binding (Dollery 1991) and should be well tolerated by elderly people.

Two published studies have examined the efficacy of lofepramine in elderly depressed patients: against amitriptyline (Jessel et al. 1981), and against dothiepin (Fairbairn et al. 1989). Both studies had relatively low drop-out rates and although Fairbairn et al. (1989) included only patients with DSM III major depressive episode, both studies used relatively appropriate outcome measures. COMP analyses only were provided, and lofepramine was found to be significantly more effective than amitriptyline and as effective as dothiepin. Analysis of side-effects showed no difference from amitriptyline but less dry mouth and drowsiness than dothiepin.

Though lofepramine thus appears to be a reasonably effective antidepressant for elderly people, these results must be viewed with some caution. In particular, there is no placebo-controlled data and no ITT analyses; doses of both lofepramine and the comparators were relatively low (with no data on plasma levels achieved); and total numbers of subjects included were small. There is also no long-term data on the efficacy of lofepramine in preventing relapse.

FLUVOXAMINE

Fluvoxamine is chemically and pharmacologically distinct from tricyclic anti-depressants and is a potent and selective inhibitor of serotonin re-uptake. Animal studies show it to be free of MAO-inhibiting and anticholinergic effects and to have negligible effects on noradrenaline re-uptake Classen et al. 1977). It is rapidly absorbed, has no active metabolites and is excreted via the kidneys with a plasma half-life of about 15 hours that is unaffected by age (Benfield and Ward 1986).

There have been three double-blind controlled comparisons between fluvox-amine and standard antidepressants in elderly patients. Only one trial (Wakelin

Table 7.2 Controlled trials of newer antidepressants in old age

	Entry criteria	Entered	Completed	Age Range	Age Mean	Drug	Dose (mg)	Duration (weeks)	Outcome measures	Analysis	Results (% responder where given)	Comments
Jessel et al. (1981)	Clin.	20	19	64–84	70.5	Lofepramine	105	4	CGI	COMP	L(72%) = A(48%)	
		19	18	65–78	68	Amitriptyline	75					
Fairbairn et al. (1989)	DSM III	30	24	68–88	77	Lofepramine	140	6	MADRS	COMP	L = D	
	MDE	32	24	65–88	77	Dothiepin	100					
Wakelin (1986)	DSM III	33	24	60–71	65	Fluvoxamine	150–300	4	HDRS	COMP	F(79%) = I(65%)	
	MAD	29	16	60–70	66	Imipramine	150–300		CGI		>P(25%)	
		14	12	60–68	64	Placebo	N/A					
Rahman et al. (1991)	DSM III	26	17	65–86	73	Fluvoxamine	100–200	6	MADRS	NR	F(64%) = D(60%)	
	MDE	26	19	61–85	75	Dothiepin	100–200		CGI			
Phanjoo et al. (1991)	DSM III	25	16	66–86	76	Fluvoxamine	100–200	6	MADRS	NR	F = M	CGI: fluoxetine superiod at 2 weeks
	MDE	25	16	66–87	77	Mianserin	40–80		CGI			
Feighner et al. (1985)	DSM III	78	41	61–90	NR	Fluoxetine	20–80	6	HDRS	ITT	F(49%) = D(48%)	
	MDE	79	31	61–90		Doxepin	50–200		CGI			
Falk et al. (1989)	DSM III	13	10	—	69	Fluoxetine	20–60	6	HDRS	ITT	F = T	Very high drop-out rate on trazodone
	MDE	12	3	—	68	Trazodone	50–400		CGI			
Altamura et al. (1989)	DSM III	13	11	NR	68.5	Fluoxetine	20	5	HDRS	COMP	F = A	Faster onset of action with amitriptyline
	MDE	15	11	NR		Amitriptyline	75					

Study	Diagnostic criteria	No. entered	No. completed	Age range	Mean age	Drug	Dose	Weeks	Scale	Analysis	Outcome
Hutchinson et al. (1991)	DSM III MDE	58 / 32	46 / 21	NR / (>65)	72 / 71.5	Paroxetine Amitriptyline	30 100	6	HDRS	COMP	P(55%) = A(59%)
Halikas (1990)	DSM III MDE	132 / 132	92 / 96	NR (>60) / NR		Paroxetine Doxepin	40 200	6	HDRS CGI	ITT	P = D (P > D on depression item)
Dorman (1992)	DSM III	29 / 28	24 / 25	NR / (>65)		Paroxetine Mianserin	30 60	6	HDRS	COMP	P(48%) > M(18%)
Dunner et al. (1992)	DSM III MDE	136 / 135	92 / 96	— / —	68 / 68	Paroxetine Doxepin	10–40 200	6	HDRS MADRS CGI	COMP	P > D (CGI) — Trend favouring paroxetine on most measures
Tiller et al. (1990)	DSM III MDE	21 / 20	13 / 13	— / —	70 / 70	Moclobemide Mianserin	150–600 30–90	4	HDRS	COMP sequential	Mo = Mi
De Vanna et al. (1990)	DSM III MDE	40 / 40	32 / 34	60–80	—	Moclobemide Mianserin	300–5000 75–125	4	HDRS	COMP	Mo = Mi
De Vanna et al. (1990)	ICD9 Endog. or neurotic	20 / 19	— / —	>60	—	Moclobemide Maprotiline	150–300 75–150	6	HDRS	COMP	Mo = Mi
Cohn et al. (1990)	DSM III MDE & BIP	161 / 80	82 / 39	63–85 / 65–82	70 / 71	Sertraline Amitriptyline	50–200 50–150	8	HDRS CGI	COMP/	COMP (CGI): S(69%) = A(64%) ITT (HDRS): A > S

Clin. = clinical; BIP = bipolar disorder; MAD = major affective disorder; NR = not recorded.

1986) incorporated a placebo group. This study included subjects ranging in age between 60 and 71 and, therefore, did not examine a representative elderly sample. Drop-out rates were relatively high in both active (fluvoxamine and imipramine) groups and the study lasted only four weeks. Clear superiority of both active drugs over placebo was demonstrated for completers. It should be noted, however, that this superiority is very much less striking if the data is subjected to ITT analysis. The studies by Rahman et al. (1991) and Phanjoo et al. (1991) compared fluvoxamine with dothiepin and mianserin respectively. Neither of these studies had a placebo group, both had similarly high drop-out rates to those in the Wakelin (1986) study, but both examined more truly elderly patients, (ages ranging up to 87), had more adequate treatment durations of 6 weeks, and used appropriate outcome measures (MADRS and CGI). Both studies found fluvoxamine to be as effective as the comparator drugs. Rahman et al. (1991) also provided adequate information about response rates, which at 64% for fluvoxamine and 60% for dothiepin are similar to those reported in studies in younger patients. Surprisingly, side-effect profiles were similar for fluvoxamine and comparators in all the studies, although Wakelin (1986) found fluvoxamine to give rise to significantly less dry mouth that imipramine.

In the context of controlled clinical trials, fluvoxamine appears to be reasonably effective and well tolerated. Comparison against placebo is, however, very limited both by small numbers and high drop-out rates, and there are no published data addressing the question of the drug's efficacy in relapse prevention.

FLUOXETINE

Like the other SSRIs currently available, fluoxetine has a novel pharmacological structure and is relatively free of cardiovascular, anticholinergic, antihistaminic and hypotensive effects (Feighner 1983). Lucas and Osborne (1986) have examined the pharmacokinetics of fluoxetine and its major active metabolite norfluoxetine in elderly depressed patients and found no alteration in elimination of the drug with age. It should however be noted that fluoxetine itself and its active metabolite norfluoxetine have extremely long elimination half lives. Three controlled comparisons between fluoxetine and established antidepressants have been published (Altamura et al. 1989; Falk et al. 1989; Feighner and Cohn 1985).

Feighner and Cohn (1985) used doxepin as comparator and relatively high doses of both drugs, with adequate treatment duration and the CGI as main outcome measure. Patients ranged widely in age and the drop-out rate was very high, approaching 50% in the fluoxetine group and exceeding it in the doxepin group. Despite the high drop-out rates, reasonable ITT response rates were seen which did not differ between the two drugs. No formal comparisons were made of emergent side-effects, but adverse experiences were the reason for drop-out in 32% of fluoxetine patients and 43% of doxepin patients. Anticholinergic side-effects were more prominent in the doxepin group, and nausea, anxiety and insomnia in the fluoxetine group. Patients in the study who responded were continued on the same drug on an open label basis for up to 48 weeks with no significant fall off in response and no emergent difference between the two drugs. The smaller study by Altamura et al. (1989) was carried out in a relatively young group (mean age 68.5 years), had a relatively short treatment period of five weeks and a fairly low dose of comparator drug (amitriptyline 75 mg). Drop-out rates were low but only COMP analyses were reported, showing the two drugs to be equivalent. Amitriptyline appeared to have a faster onset of action, though this was not apparent for biological symptoms and presumably reflected the ability of amitriptyline to relieve anxiety and insomnia. Severity and frequency of side-effects tended to be lower in the fluoxetine group, the difference reaching statistical significance for dry mouth. There was also a significant difference in weight change through the trial with amitriptyline-treated patients showing significant weight gain.

Falk et al. (1989) compared fluoxetine and trazodone in variable doses for six weeks of active treatment. Unfortunately, only 10/14 patients on fluoxetine and 3/13 on trazodone completed the study; these numbers were insufficient for very meaningful statistical evaluation of efficacy, though significantly fewer drop-outs and more responders were found in the fluoxetine group. The only statistically significant differences in side-effects were more frequent constipation on trazodone and more insomnia on fluoxetine.

On the basis of these studies, fluoxetine appears to have a different side-effect profile from tricyclic antidepressants and, though the lack of placebo-controlled data must be borne in mind, to be comparable in efficacy with some evidence of ability to prevent relapse.

PAROXETINE

Paroxetine is a highly selective serotonin re-uptake inhibitor which is effectively absorbed and extensively (95%) protein bound, with a complex metabolic pathway of oxidation, methylation and conjugation prior to excretion in the urine (Kaye et al. 1989). The plasma half-life is approximately 24 hours but varies widely, with some evidence of increased plasma half-life in the elderly (Kaye et al. 1989).

Three controlled comparisons with established antidepressants in elderly patients have been published. Two (Dunner et al. 1992; Hutchinson et al. 1991) have appeared as full-length papers, the other (Dorman 1990) presenting limited data in a paper focusing on sleep parameters. Dunner et al. (1992), comparing paroxetine with doxepin, had a large sample size but a low mean age. Both drugs were administered in relatively high doses over six weeks and were found to be equivalent in efficacy, though paroxetine had a larger effect than doxepin on the physician-rated clinical global impression and on the depressed mood item of the HDRS. Dorman (1990), in a small study comparing paroxetine 30 mg with a relatively low dose of mianserin in a patient population unde-fined by mean age, found paroxetine to be superior to mianserin, although this finding must be viewed with some caution since only COMP analysis was reported and, though the response rate in the paroxetine group (48%) was reasonable, that in the mianserin group (18%) was very low. Hutchinson et al. (1991) compared paroxetine with amitriptyline in a relatively young (mean age 72) elderly group over six weeks. Drop-out rates were reasonable and, in a COMP only analysis, the two drugs were found to be equally effective. All three studies showed a tendency for more anticholinergic side-effects with comparator drugs than paroxetine. Dunner et al. (1992) reported significantly more frequent dry mouth, somnolence, headache, confusion and constipation with doxepin, but more diarrhoea and nausea with paroxetine. Similarly, Hutchinson et al. (1991) reported that anticholinergic effects overall were more frequent with amitriptyline than with paroxetine.

Paroxetine thus appears to be of at least equal efficacy to comparator drugs with some suggestion of superiority, though the overall response rate to paroxetine was no higher than might be expected. Its side-effect profile in elderly patients closely resembles that which would be predicted from *in vitro* studies and data from younger patients. These conclusions would, of course, be much strengthened by pacebo-controlled trial data, and no comment can be made as to the efficacy of paroxetine in preventing depressive relapse in old age.

SERTRALINE

Sertraline is a specific serotonin re-uptake inhibitor unrelated chemically to other Saris and relatively free of anticholinergic, antihistaminic and adverse cardiovascular side-effects (Doogan and Caillard 1988). Pharmacokinetic studies (Invicta Pharmaceuticals, data on file) suggest that in elderly volunteers, the pharmacokinetics of sertraline are similar to those in younger subjects. Its major metabolite, desmethylsertraline, is found in higher concentrations in elderly subjects. The plasma half-life of sertraline in these elderly volunteers was 21.6 hours and that of desmethylsertraline 83.7 hours. Three out of twenty volunteers in an open study had to discontinue sertraline because of side-effects such as nausea, insomnia and dizziness. Comparison of the effects of sertraline and mianserin on psychomotor performance in elderly volunteers showed sertraline (at doses up to 200 mg daily) to have a generally neutral psychomotor profile (Hindmarch et al. 990) with significant improvement in vigilance compared with placebo (Hindmarch and Bhatti 1988).

The only controlled study of sertraline in elderly patients is a comparison with amitriptyline (Cohn et al. 1990). This study did not include a placebo group and, though the sample examined was relatively large, the completer rate in both sertraline and amitriptyline groups was less than 50%. While the age range was wide, the mean was relatively low. Both the doses of drugs used and the duration of the trial were adequate to allow beneficial effects to emerge. The overall analysis showed equivalent efficacy for completers, though the ITT analysis indicated some superiority for amitriptyline over sertraline in magnitude of change in the HDRS. The latter finding may be due at least in part to greater responsiveness of the anxiety and sleep items of this scale to the more sedating antidepressant. Anticholinergic side-effects were significantly commoner in the amitriptyline-treated group and gastrointestinal ones in the sertraline group, with similar side-effect-related withdrawal rates (28% on sertraline subjects and 35% on amitriptyline). There was also a modest but statistically significant difference in weight change between the groups, amitriptyline being associated with weight gain and sertraline with weight loss. Patients achieving satisfactory response in the double-blind study continued on the same therapy for an additional 16-week period with efficacy assessments at 12 and 24 weeks indicating no diminution in response from that at 8 weeks (Invicta Pharmaceuticals, data on file).

Sertraline thus appears reasonably well tolerated by elderly patients with modest evidence for efficacy in relapse prevention. However, the high withdrawal rate and lack of placebo control limit the confidence that can be placed in these results.

MOCLOBEMIDE

Moclobemide, a benzamide derivative, is a recently introduced, short-acting, reversible, selective inhibitor of monoamine-oxidase A (Da Prada et al. 1989) which can be taken without dietary restrictions except the avoidance of very excessive quantities of tyramine-containing foods. Its pharmacokinetics are very similar in younger and elderly subjects (Maguire et al. 1991). Pooled clinical trial data show it to be as effective and, unlike its tricyclic comparators, as well tolerated in elderly as in younger depressed subjects (Angst and Stabl 1992). Three small clinical trials in elderly subjects have been published to date; each involves only COMP analyses and none contains a placebo group. De Vanna et al. (1990), in a brief report from two studies, found moclobemide to be as effective as both mianserin and maprotiline. Tiller et al. (1990), using a sequential analysis design, also found no significant difference in efficacy between moclobemide and mianserin.

The published data currently available is clearly inadequate to form definite conclusions about the use of moclobemide in elderly depressed patients. The results of trials against placebo and in relapse prevention in elderly subjects are to be awaited with interest.

HOW STRONG IS THE CASE FOR USING NEWER ANTIDEPRESSANTS IN ELDERLY PATIENTS?

All the antidepressant drugs reviewed above appear to be effective in 50–60% of depressed elderly patients, suggesting that there is no clear difference in efficacy between them and their tricyclic predecessors. The almost complete absence of placebo-controlled data remains a major problem as does the severe lack of long-term efficacy data, which are of particular importance in the context of a disease as frequently recurring as depression in old age (see Chapter 8). No single drug emerges as clearly superior to the others on the basis of the evidence reviewed above, although paroxetine may be claimed to have a slight edge in terms of numbers of patients studied and evidence from two or three studies of superiority over comparator drug.

The new generation of antidepressant drugs do, however, represent a modest step forward in the treatment of depression in elderly patients and may reasonably be seen as drugs of first choice. Their advantage lies not in greater clinical trial efficacy but in the fact that they have fewer contraindications and a less disabling side-effect profile, which may enable a higher proportion of the many depressed elderly patients in the real world who would not be eligible for entry into controlled clinical trials to be treated effectively. Further evidence in terms of placebo-controlled efficacy and long-term relapse prevention is clearly needed. This will be aided in the next generation of clinical trials by critical cost–benefit appraisal (Maynard 1993) in which the impact on health services of poor compliance and adverse drug effects can be weighed up against that of drug cost.

PHARMACOLOGICAL STRATEGIES FOR RESISTANT DEPRESSION IN OLD AGE

As has been discussed above, antidepressant drugs offer no guarantee of response in elderly patients, any more than is the case for depression in younger subjects. In patients failing to respond, full review, including assessment of the appropriateness and adequacy (in terms of dosage, duration and compliance) of any treatment trial should be undertaken. The use of electroconvulsive therapy and of specific psychological approaches (discussed below) should also be considered.

Several drug combination treatments (such as tricyclic–MAOI combinations, the addition of tri-iodothyronine and the co-administration of tricyclic antidepressants and neuroleptics) have been proposed and to a limited extent evaluated in younger patients; these are reviewed by Katona (1991). These treatment manoeuvres have, however, received no evaluation in elderly subjects and are in any case likely to be relatively hazardous.

Georgotas et al. (1983) have, however, noted that 65% of elderly patients failing to respond to tricyclic antidepressants recovered during an open trial of phenelzine. Another treatment option is the addition of lithium, which is probably the best-evaluated pharmacological strategy in younger antidepressant-resistant patients (Austin et al. 1991; Katona 1991). Kushnir (1986) reported the benefit of lithium augmentation in a small open series of five elderly physically ill patients. In a retrospective analysis of a consecutive series of elderly depressed patients, Finch and Katona (1989) demonstrated a clinically useful response to lithium augmentation in 6/9 patients, with maintained benefit for up to 18 months. Similar acute responses have been noted by Lafferman et al. (1988) with

7/14 subjects showing complete remission and a further three a partial response. A larger retrospective series by Bekker et al. (1990) reported complete response to lithium augmentation in 15/43, with symptomatic improvement in another 15. Lithium augmentation thus appears the best-documented pharmacological option for refractory depression in old age. It must, however, be borne in mind that placebo-controlled evaluation in the elderly is as yet lacking. Furthermore, as reviewed by Katona and Finch (1990) and attested to by all the studies referred to here, neurological side-effects to lithium are common in the elderly and lithium augmentation must be carried out cautiously. Since lithium toxicity may occur at relatively low serum levels in the elderly, initial dose of lithium should be low (100–200 mg/day) with gradual dosage titration to achieve blood levels within a downward-adjusted therapeutic range (0.4–0.8 mmol/l).

ELECTROCONVULSIVE THERAPY

Electroconvulsive therapy (ECT) is an important treatment option in the more severe depressive illnesses of old age. As will be reviewed below, it not only appears to be relatively safe (when compared with tricyclic antidepressants or with withholding treatment altogether), but may even be more effective in the elderly than in the younger depressed patient. Since elderly depressed patients are more likely than their younger counterparts to be physically frail and to be taking a large number of drugs, the administration of ECT is none the less a cause for considerable concern. In this chapter, the use of ECT in the elderly will be considered in terms of the following broad considerations, after the example of the excellent review by Benbow (1989). How likely are elderly patients with depression to respond to ECT? What physical and neuropsychological problems are likely to be encountered? Which elderly depressed patients are most likely to respond to the treatment? What is the optimal ECT procedure (type of stimulus, electrode placement, pre-medication, etc.) for elderly patients? What are the contraindications to ECT in old age?

WHAT PROPORTION OF ELDERLY DEPRESSED PATIENTS RESPOND TO ECT?

Two early studies (Gold and Chiarella 1944; Hobson 1953) reported higher response rates in older than in younger patients, though the former study did not include patients aged over 60 and the latter used 40 as its age cut-off. Unfortunately, none of the studies comparing ECT with sham ECT under blind controlled conditions (reviewed by Freeman 1993) contained sufficient subjects aged over 65 to allow separate analyses of the elderly group. There have, however, been several non-blind evaluations of ECT in specifically elderly subjects. The most comprehensive review of these studies was carried out by Mulsant et al. (1991), who identified 1025 patients from 14 studies. Twelve of them gave sufficient details to allow subjects to be allocated into those with good, intermediate and poor outcomes. Out of the 659 patients who were amenable to such analysis, 410 (62%) had good outcome, 140 (21%) intermediate outcome and 109 (17%) poor outcome. Mulsant et al. also reported the findings of their own study of 40 elderly patients: 23 of these had a good outcome, 6 an intermediate outcome and 9 a poor outcome. When these figures are added to the total from earlier studies, all the percentages remain unchanged. It is thus clear that at least 80% of elderly patients receiving ECT can be expected to have a useful clinical response with full or nearly full recovery in almost two-thirds. This is very similar to the optimum response rate that might be expected in younger patients and is considerably higher than the response rate in the controlled trials reviewed by Freeman (1993). Similar results have recently been reported by Wilkinson (1993), who examined response to ECT in a naturalistic sample of patients divided into age bands and found significantly better responses in the over-65s. These studies provide at least some support for the conclusion by Weiner (1982) that older people 'may actually have a better therapeutic response to ECT'.

THE SAFETY OF ECT IN OLD AGE

Benbow (1989) provides a comprehensive review of physical problems encountered by elderly people receiving ECT. Rare complications can include vertebral fracture, bladder rupture, cerebral haemorrhage and myocardial infarction. Chest infections have also been reported as infrequent complications by Gaspar and Samarasinghe (1982), Fraser and Glass (1980) and Karlinsky and Shulman (1984). Two of the 40 patients treated by Mulsant et al. (1991) experienced symptomatic vertebral compression fractures. Serious adverse events in elderly patients receiving ECT are much more likely in those in poor physical (and particularly cardiovascular) health (Burke et al. 1985).

Cognitive side-effects are a particular problem in the elderly. The most important of these are post-ECT delirious states and longer-lasting anterograde and retrograde memory impairment. Mulsant et al. (1991) reported clinically significant confusion in 13 out of 40 (31%) of their subjects, which in some patients (10%) was still present 10–17 days after the end of the course of ECT. Not surprisingly, post-ECT confusion was commoner in subjects with organic mood disorders than in those with pure depressive illnesses. Figiel et al. (1990), in a prospective study of 36 elderly depressed patients undergoing ECT, found that prolonged delirium occurred in (17%). CT or MRI scan in the patients who became delirious revealed that all 6 had abnormalities in the caudate nucleus (hyperintensities on MRI and hypodensity on CT). Interpretation of these data is difficult, since none of the patients received scans prior to the course of ECT, and patients not becoming delirious did not receive post-ECT scans. The authors also point out that similar basal ganglia changes are seen in a proportion of healthy elderly controls. They suggest that pre-existing subcortical abnormalities may represent a marker for vulnerability to post-ECT delirium, rather than reflecting ECT-induced brain damage. These conclusions are in keeping with the report by

Raskind (1984) of a post-mortem examination of the brain of an 89-year-old woman. Despite more than 1000 ECT treatments, her brain showed no evidence of damage.

Memory deficits frequently occur in elderly patients receiving ECT. The review by Benbow (1989) concludes that anterograde amnesia fades gradually after completion of a cure of ECT, resolving completely within six months. Retrograde amnesia also shrinks gradually following the end of a course of ECT, leaving permanent memory loss only for events in the week or two prior to the start of treatment. The study by Fraser and Glass (1980) found striking improvements in memory from quite impaired pre-treatment baselines in 20 elderly depressed patients receiving ECT. Scores remained below normal until after the end of the course of ECT, but by three weeks after treatment all scores were well within one standard deviation of age-related norms. Very similar findings have recently been reported by Stoudemire et al. (1991), who reported improvements in cognitive impairment both in elderly depressed patients treated with ECT and in a group treated with tricyclic antidepressants.

As well as giving rise to organic cognitive impairment, ECT may cause considerable subjective anxiety, both in patients themselves and in their relatives. Wilkinson (1993) reports an unpublished study by Heggs in which 11 elderly patients receiving ECT were rated for severity and foci of anxiety before and after a course of ECT and after discharge. In general, anxiety levels fell with treatment, but in six of the nine patients who experienced an overall fall in anxiety levels, this was preceded by an increase in anxiety after the third or fourth treatment. Most frequent foci of anxiety before treatment were fear of brain damage and of side-effects. After ECT, anxiety was most often focused on memory loss, the use of anaesthetics, and not knowing what would happen. At follow-up, the only remaining areas of anxiety concerned the use of anaesthetic and the memory of anticipating ECT the night before each treatment. Three of the patients stated after discharge that they would not be willing to receive ECT again. Wilkinson concluded that there was an important role for education of patients and their relatives in the nature of ECT. His practice is to use a videotape as the main means of such education.

PREDICTORS OF RESPONSE TO ECT

Hobson (1953) and Carney et al. (1965) have published rating scales for predicting response to ECT in age-unselected subjects. In both cases, the critical clinical features were similar but not identical to those distinguishing endogenous from neurotic depression. Katona et al. (1987) provided some validation for the Carney et al. (1965) scale in a sample including a number of elderly patients, but the much larger Northwick Park ECT study (Johnstone et al. 1980) failed to validate the scale. Both this study and the Leicester ECT control trial (Brandon et al. 1984) found that the most consistent predictors of response to ECT were delusions and psychomotor retardation.

Three studies restricted to elderly patients have compared clinical features in those with a good response and those with poor outcome. Gaspar and Samarisinghe (1982) emphasised the importance of psychotic depression with nihilistic, guilty or hypochondriacal delusions as indications for using ECT as treatment of first choice in elderly depressed patients. Fraser and Glass (1980) examined individual items of the HDRS and found that patients with good outcome had more severe depressed mood and also showed higher scores on HDRS items for guilt, agitation, overall severity and (in contrast with Hobson 1953 and Carney et al. 1965) psychic anxiety. They also had less chronic illnesses. In a similar retrospective study, Magni et al. (1988) examined the case records of 30 consecutive elderly patients meeting DSM III criteria for major depression and treated with ECT, of whom 19 had a good outcome and 11 a poor outcome. Poor outcome was associated with a more chronic depressive illness and with the presence of coexistent physical illness. Non-responders were also significantly less likely to have experienced adverse life events before the onset of their depression.

Wilkinson (1993) concludes that in elderly subjects the presence of retardation, delusions of guilt or suicidal intent suggest that ECT is almost certainly going to be successful. Given the evidence that depression cannot be classified in the same way in old age as it can in younger people, and in particular that the endogenous/neurotic distinction does not appear to hold its validity in old age (see Chapter 1), it is unlikely that scales derived in younger samples (Carney et al. 1965; Hobson 1953) would have similar predictive power in elderly subjects. Thus Wilkinson's (1993) brief set of predictive criteria are probably the most useful for routine clinical practice.

THE ADMINISTRATION OF ECT IN OLD AGE

The practice of using routine atropine premedication in patients receiving ECT has fallen out of favour because the risks associated with anticholinergic medication probably outweigh those of unprotected vagal stimulation. Sommer et al. (1989) carried out a formal comparison in an elderly sample between premedication with atropine and with glycopyrrolate (an anticholinergic drug which does not normally cross the bloody–brain barrier). No significant difference in outcome (in terms of memory dysfunction or antidepressant response) were found between the two groups, although, surprisingly, there was a consistent trend for the glycopyrrolate group to show more marked cognitive impairment. The authors suggest that because of the increased permeability of the blood–brain barrier induced by ECT, the glycopyrrolate might in fact be acting centrally after all. They propose that an alternative strategy might be to administer cholinomimetic agents prior to ECT, quoting a preliminary study in younger patients (Levin et al. 1987) with promising results. In view of the findings cited above that ECT-induced memory changes are outweighed by the memory ameliorating effects of recovery from depression, this issue may in any case not be as important as previously thought.

There have been no recent studies looking systematically at choice of anaesthetic or muscle relaxant in elderly patients receiving ECT, and no study restricted to elderly patients of different electrical modalities (sinewave vs brief pulse, threshold vs suprathreshold, etc). The question of unilateral electrode placement (UNI) vs bilateral (BI) has, however, been examined in elderly subjects. Fraser and Glass (1978) studied nine elderly patients treated alternately with UNI and BI electrode placement, using threshold bidirectional pulse stimuli. BI was associated with much longer recovery times (in terms of consciousness, restoration and orientation). Recovery times for both UNI and BI were longer than would be expected in a younger population, the difference being more marked for BI placement. Another study by Fraser and Glass (1980) has shown that UNI was associated with markedly fewer side-effects, but no diminution in clinical efficacy.

The reviews by Benbow (1989) and Wilkinson (1993) both conclude that, in elderly patients, UNI should be used in the first instance. Wilkinson (1993) reports that in a retrospective survey of his own clinical experience of ECT, BI was not associated with any decrease in number of treatments given. He concedes that in patients apparently not responding to UNI, the switch to BI is a reasonable clinical step after 4–6 applications. Wilkinson (1993) also strongly favours the use of substantially suprathreshold stimuli, particularly in patients receiving UNI. This approach, most prominently championed by Weiner's group (Weiner et al. 1986), may be particularly important in the elderly, since age is associated with increased seizure threshold (Sackeim et al. 1987). The use of specific techniques to increase the 'efficiency' of ECT, such as dose titration (Sackeim et al. 1986), and the placement of the ECT electrodes bifrontally (Letemendia et al. 1993) have not been evaluated in an exclusively elderly sample.

CONTRAINDICATIONS TO ECT IN OLD AGE

There are no absolute contraindications to ECT apart from the absence of a head on which to place the electrodes. Wilkinson (1993) emphasises the need to weigh up the relative risks of ECT against those of alternative treatments or of the withholding of treatment altogether. Great caution must be used in patients recovering from crescendo angina, recent myocardial infarction or stroke and in those with raised intracranial pressure. Safety can, however, be maximised by good liaison between psychiatrist and anaesthetist and by a policy of considering ECT relatively early, particularly in patients with concurrent physical illness. Failure to do so leads all too frequently to the hopeless situation of a patient whose depression, which might earlier have been successfully treated with ECT, has led to dehydration and thence to irreversible renal failure.

PSYCHOLOGICAL APPROACHES TO THE TREATMENT OF DEPRESSION IN OLD AGE

Psychological treatments for depression can broadly be divided into those dependent upon the acquisition of psychodynamic insights; those focusing on abnormal cognitive processes; and those primarily attempting to modify behaviour. All these approaches have been applied with at least some success in elderly depressed subjects, but neither their clinical use nor their evaluation has been as widespread as in younger depressed subjects. As Morris and Morris (1991) point out, the reluctance to use psychological approaches is in large part a legacy of the Freudian view that elderly people lack the capacity for mental change that is necessary to engage in therapy. Though age-related changes in mental function- ing undoubtedly do necessitate modifications of the psychological techniques for treating depression, it is becoming increasingly recognised that they do not render them entirely impractical. In particular, Morris and Morris (1991) suggest the importance of making the goals of therapy more explicit, to maintain a flexible approach with the setting of concrete and realistic goals, and to be aware of the genuine social and physical limitations that elderly patients are likely to have. Both behavioural (Gallagher 1981) and cognitive (Emery 1981) therapies have been specifically modified for use in the elderly with these principles in mind. In both cases, patients receive a booklet explaining the rationale of treatment and suggesting that they keep a diary monitoring their mood and behaviour or thinking.

The evaluation of such modified psychological treatments remains difficult. Mintz et al. (1981) have reviewed the research aspects of psychotherapy with depressed elderly patients, and conclude that the main difficulties include the confounding effects of concurrent physical illness and the possible influence of the therapist being younger than the patient. They also point out that the majority of evaluative studies of psychological treatments in depression have specifically excluded elderly people, and that even those that do include elderly subjects have failed to distinguish between the young-old and the old-old. A further problem in the critical evaluation of these studies is that in many cases the primary outcome measure is the Beck Depression Inventory (BDI; Beck et al. 1961), which may be expected to change preferentially in treatment aimed at changing the depressive cognitions which form a large part of the scale's content. Mintz et al. (1981) also point out that in view of the relatively high risk involved in physical treatment of elderly frail patients, the potential benefits of psychological treatments (which may be expected not to have physical side-effects) are particularly high. Such treatments are thus eminently worthy of rigorous evaluation.

INSIGHT THERAPIES

The Freudian model of psychological development and of psychoanalysis is parti- cularly difficult to apply to elderly subjects both because of its focus on events in early childhood and, as referred to earlier, because of Freud's own strongly held view that elderly people lack the capacity for psychodynamic change. Kelleher (1992) points out that Jung's psychodynamic model, in contrast to that of Freud, laid an emphasis on continuing development throughout the life cycle and in particular identified developmental tasks specific to middle and old age. Not only is the Jungian view therefore more positive about aging, but it also provides a much clearer framework for offering dynamic psychotherapy to older people, including those with depression. Kelleher (1992) provides a lucid summary of this framework. In the second half of life, once social goals and the begetting of children are completed, the legitimate focus of psychological development becomes one of acquiring personal wholeness. According to this model, elderly people with depression experience, as their primary problem, an absence of meaning in their lives. The psychotherapeutic task is, therefore, to carry out a life review in order to enable them to value more appropriately what they have done in their lives.

Jungian psychotherapy has not received formal evaluation in the context of depression in old age. Indeed, the main evaluations of insight therapies in elderly depressed patients have come through their use as controls for the cognitive and behavioural treatments to be discussed later in this chapter (see Table 7.3). Steer et al. (1984) compared the efficacy of psychodynamic group therapy against that of a mixture of cognitive and behavioural therapy in a total of 53 patients. The treatments were found to be roughly equivalent, with slight superiority shown for the cognitive–behavioural treatment in BDI scores but not on other measures of depression. Similarly, a series of studies by Gallagher's group (Gallagher and Thompson 1982, 1983; Thompson et al. 1987) compared the effectiveness of cognitive therapy, behaviour therapy and 'brief relational/insight psychotherapy'. All these studies showed the treatments to be roughly equivalent in short-term efficacy although the earliest study (Gallagher and Thompson 1982) found that improvement was less well sustained with relational/insight psychotherapy than with cognitive or behaviour therapy.

A further approach, described by Viney et al. (1990), is the application of the personal construct therapy developed by Kelly (1955) to elderly subjects. In particular, Viney et al. (1990) suggest that exploring and modifying the ways that elderly people make sense of the personal and social losses that old age brings may have considerable therapeutic benefit. Personal construct therapy has not, however, received controlled evaluation against other treatment modalities or control conditions in elderly depressed patients.

Despite the relative lack of objective evidence for the efficacy of formally administered insight therapies in elderly depressed patients, psychodynamic insight may nonetheless be useful in routine psychiatric work with elderly patients even where they have significant cognitive impairment as well as depression. Treliving (1989) has provided a fascinating account of her practice of routinely eliciting dreams from all the patients she admitted to an acute assessment ward for elderly people with functional psychiatric illness. In her view, Freudian perspectives were particularly useful in understanding such patients' frequent preoccupation with their bowel habits. Similarly, Hartman and Lazarus (1992) suggest that Freudian insights may be particularly relevant to the

Table 7.3 Controlled trials of cognitive and behavioural treatments for depression in old age (adapted from Morris and Morris 1991)

Authors	Type of therapy	Cell size	Length (weeks)	Average age (yr)	Outcome
Gallagher and Thompson (1982)	Cognitive	10	12		
	Behavioural	10	12	68.3	Equivalent
	Psychotherapy	10	12		
Gallagher and Thompson (1983)	Behavioural	10	12	66.0	
	Psychotherapy	10	12	69.0	Equivalent
Steuer et al. (1984)	Cognitive	26	37.5	66.0	
	Psychodynamic	27	37.5		Cog > Dynamic on BDI
Beutler et al. (1987)	Cognitive and placebo	16	20		
	Cognitive and alprazolam	13	20	70.7	
	Placebo and support	15	20		Active treatments equivalent; all > control
	Alprazolam and support	12	20		
Thompson et al. (1987)	Cognitive	27	20	66.9	
	Behavioural	25	20	67.1	
	Psychodynamic	24	20	66.7	Active treatments equivalent; all > control
	Delayed treatment	19		67.6	
Zerhusen et al. (1991)	Group cognitive	20	10		
	Music			77.0	
	Routine nursing care				Cognitive > other groups
Campbell et al. (1992)	Cognitive	34	8	64–82 (range)	
	Group craft activities				Cognitive > craft, control
	Waiting list controls				

understanding of the conflicts, losses and disappointments of elderly depressed patients.

COGNITIVE THERAPY

Lovestone (1993) provides a useful summary of the concepts integral to cognitive therapy for depression. Three types of abnormal thinking are seen as underpinning the development and maintenance of depression. These are the cognitive triad (the patient's negative view of him/herself as useless, the future as bleak and the outside world as hostile); negative schemata (in which automatic negative thoughts result in events being interpreted in an exclusively negative way); and faulty information processing (in which dysfunctional thought patterns, such as overgeneralisation and misattribution, result in further negative interpretations of events). The essence of cognitive therapy is to use 'collaborative empiricism' to encourage logical, rational thinking and thereby to recognise the link between cognitive patterns and abnormal mood; to monitor negative thought and schemata and dysfunctional information processing; and to challenge their validity. Lam and Power (1991) have confirmed a similar link between dysfunctional attitudes (or negative cognition) and depression in elderly subjects to that found in younger adults.

Cognitive therapy has been very extensively evaluated in the treatment of younger depressed patients. There is consistent evidence that, in non-psychotic subjects, it is equivalent in efficacy to antidepressant treatment and may give rise to longer-lasting benefits. Perhaps more important, there is also consistent evidence that the combination of antidepressant drugs and cognitive therapy is therapeutically superior to either treatment in isolation (Blackburn et al. 1981)

Cognitive therapy has also undergone relatively stringent testing in elderly subjects (see Table 7.3). Morris and Morris (1991) review a total of five studies in which cognitive psychotherapy is compared with behavioural or psychodynamic treatments and in one case (Beutler et al. 1987) also with the benzodiazepine drug alprazolam. In general, these studies show the various treatments evaluated to be roughly equivalent. The study by Beutler et al. (1987) is particularly important since its incorporation of a drug treatment comparison group also allowed the inclusion of a small number of subjects on placebo who showed significantly less improvement than any of the active treatment groups.

Interestingly, Marmar et al. (1989) found that good outcome following cognitive therapy in elderly patients was significantly associated with the degree to which (in assessments carried out prior to the onset of treatment) patients felt committed to the treatment and were judged to be able to develop new insights. The latter findings suggest that the distinction between cognitive and insight or dynamic psychotherapies is perhaps more apparent than real.

Two more recent trials (Campbell 1992; Zerhusen et al. 1991) evaluated cognitive therapy as delivered to elderly depressed patients in a group setting by nurses. Zerhusen et al. (1991) studied 60 depressed nursing home residents allocated randomly to cognitive therapy, music therapy and routine nursing care over a ten-week period. Beck Depression Scores decreased substantially in the cognitive group but not in the music therapy or control group. Campbell (1992) compared the effects of random allocation to cognitive therapy and group craft activities as well as examining a cohort of matched waiting list controls in subjects aged between 64 and 82 and fulfilling DSM IIIR criteria for depression. At the end of eight weeks, during which the cognitive therapy group kept daily diaries and received nursing intervention aimed at reinforcing positive thought patterns, Self-Rated Depression Scores (Zung 1965) had reduced significantly in the cognitive group and slightly in the craft group but not at all in the controls.

The evidence is thus quite consistent that cognitive therapy does result in measurable and (in those studies that have examined it) relatively sustained improvements in depression. The crucial issues of cost effectiveness and of relative efficacy against antidepressant drugs are, however, yet to be addressed.

BEHAVIOURAL THERAPIES

The rationale for behavioural treatments for depression in old age are well summarised by Morris and Morris (1991). The behavioural approach conceptualises depression as an extinction phenomenon if social reinforcement of normal behaviour is reduced or ceases. Its alleviation is dependent on the development of alternative reinforcers. Behavioural therapy attempts to restore a schedule of positive reinforcers, thereby reinstating previous positive behaviour patterns and/or establishing new activities. In conjunction with this, patients are encouraged, with the aid of specific skills such as time management and relaxation training, to plan their daily activities and to keep track of the relationship between pleasurable activity and positive mood. In particular, an attempt is made to substitute still feasible activities for those that patients' can no longer do because of their physical handicaps. Whereas long walks may no longer be possible, for example, excursions by car or public transport may provide a pleasurable alternative.

The major studies evaluating behavioural therapy in elderly depressed patients have involved systematic comparisons with cognitive therapy and are summarised with them in Table 7.3. In general, behavioural therapy is of similar efficacy to cognitive therapy with similar though limited evidence of maintained therapeutic benefit. As with cognitive therapy, controlled comparisons with antidepressant drugs have yet to be carried out.

OTHER PSYCHOLOGICAL APPROACHES

Several other psychological treatments have been proposed as potentially useful in elderly depressed subjects. In general, these have received even less formal evaluation than the insight, cognitive and behavioural approaches outlined above. Morris and Morris (1991) emphasise the potential benefits of reminiscence therapy, problem solving and skills training. Family therapy, though also not as yet subjected to formal testing in the context of depression in old age, may be crucial in modifying 'maintenance factors' that make recovery from depression impossible. Benbow et al. (1990) have provided a detailed description of a family clinic in the context of an old age psychiatry service, and include detailed case material on work with the families of depressed patients. A short paper by McNeil et al. (1991) reported the formal evaluation of experimenter-accompanied walking compared with increased social contact (visits by an undergraduate student) and waiting list control. BDI scores reduced significantly in both active treatment conditions. Somatic symptoms, however, only decreased significantly in the exercise group.

There is no shortage of potentially useful psychological treatments for depression in old age and a clear need for more adequate evaluation of each of them. Meanwhile, cognitive therapy is probably the most feasible and best-evaluated treatment approach. Formal cognitive or behavioural treatments are useful adjuncts or even alternatives to conventional antidepressant treatment. As is the case with the psychodynamic approach, cognitive or behavioural insights may also be therapeutically valuable in many patients not receiving formal psychological treatment.

CONCLUSIONS

The grounds for therapeutic optimism in managing older depressed patients are considerable, despite the particular challenges to be met in treating such a vulnerable group. Antidepressant drugs have been relatively rigorously evaluated and found to be effective in the more severely ill patients and under controlled conditions. The utility of antidepressants in the milder depressions encountered in primary care has yet to be properly evaluated. Though newer antidepressants have not been shown to have an overwhelming advantage, their relative safety and the lack of associated cognitive impairment may justify their use as first-choice drugs in an elderly population. Electroconvulsive therapy also has a well-established role in the severe depressions of old age, and has a remarkably good profile in terms both of safety and efficacy. Even in apparently treatment resistant cases, the response to more aggressive treatment approaches can be gratifying and not necessarily associated with excessive hazard.

Psychological techniques are probably of far greater potential in the elderly than their relatively limited formal evaluation to date suggests. The move away from an 'ageist' perspective, in which elderly depressed patients are seen as too rigid to achieve psychological change, is strongly to be welcomed. Finally, the principles of holistic management (which are almost invariably neglected in formal treatment evaluations), the role of multidisciplinary teamwork and the importance of other family members in the treatment alliance should not be forgotten.

REFERENCES

Altamura AC, Percudani M, Guercetti G and Invernizzi G (1989) Efficacy and tolerability of fluoxetine in the elderly: a double-blind study versus amitrityline. *International Clinical Psychopharmacology* 4, 103-6.

American Psychiatric Association (1980) *Diagnostic and Statistical Manual of Mental Disorders* (3rd edn). Washington, American Psychiatric Association.

American Psychiatric Association (1987) *Diagnostic and Statistical Manual of Mental Disorders* (3rd edn, revised). Washington, American Psychiatric Association.

Angst J and Stabl M (1992) Efficacy of moclobemide in different patient groups: a meta-analysis of studies. *Psychopharmacology* 106, S109-13.

Austin M-PV, Souza FGM and Goodwin GM (1991) Lithium augmentation in antidepressant-resistant patients. A quantitative analysis. *British Journal of Psychiatry* 159, 510-14.

Beck AT, Ward CH, Mendelson M et al. (1961) An inventory for measuring depression. *Archives of General Psychiatry* 159, 510-14.

Bekker FM, van Marwijk HWJ, Nolen WA et al. (1990) Lithium bij de behandeling van depressieve bejaarden. *Nederland Tijdschrift Geneeskden* 134, 442-5.

Benbow SM (1989) The role of electroconvulsive therapy in the treatment of depressive illness in old age. *British Journal of Psychiatry* 155, 147-52.

Benbow S, Egan G, Marriott A et al. (1990) Using the family life cycle with later life families. *Journal of Family Therapy* 12, 321-40.

Benfield P and Ward A (1986) Fluvoxamine: a review of its pharmacodynamic and pharmacokinetic properties and therapeutic efficacy in depressive illness. *Drugs* 32, 313-4.

Beutler LE, Scogin F, Kirkish P et al. (1987) Group cognitive therapy and alprazolam in the treatment of depression in older adults. *Journal of Consulting and Clinical Psychology* 55, 550-6.

Blackburn IM, Bishop S, Glen AIM et al. (1981) The efficacy of cognitive therapy in depression: a treatment trial using cognitive therapy and pharmacotherapy, each alone and in combination. *British Journal of Psychiatry* 139, 181-9.

Blanchard MR, Waterreus A and Mann AH (1994) Depression amongst older people within the community: the effect of intervention. *British Journal of Psychiatry*, in press.

Branconnier RJ, Cole JO, Ghasvinian S et al. (1982) Treating the depressed elderly patient: the comparative behavioural pharmacology of mianserin and amitriptyline. In Costa E and Racagni G (eds) *Typical and Atypical Antidepressants: Clinical Practice*. New York, Raven Press.

Brandon S, Cowley P, McDonald C et al. (1984) Electroconvulsive therapy: results in depressive illness from the Leicestershire trial. *British Medical Journal* 288, 22-5.

Burke WJ, Rutherford JL, Zorumski CF et al. (1985) Electroconvulsive therapy and the elderly. *Comprehensive Psychiatry* 26, 480-6.

Campbell AJ (1991) Drug treatment as a cause of fall in old age: a review of offending agents. *Drugs and Aging* 1, 289-302.

Campbell JM (1992) Treating depression in well older adults: use of diaries in cognitive therapy. *Issues in Mental Health Nursing* 13, 19-29.

Carney MWP, Roth M and Garside RF (1965) The diagnosis of depressive syndromes and the prediction of ECT response. *British Journal of Psychiatry* 111, 659-74.

Classen V, Davies JE, Hertting G et al. (1977) Fluvoxamine: a specific 5-hydroxytryptamine uptake inhibitor. *British Journal of Pharmacology* 60, 505-16.

Cohn CK, Shrivastava R, Mendels J et al. (1990) Double-blind, multicenter comparison of sertraline and amitriptyline in elderly depressed patients. *Journal of Clinical Psychiatry* 51, 28-33.

Copeland JR, Davidson IA, Dewey ME et al. (1992) Alzheimer's Disease, other dementia, depression and pseudodementia: prevalence, incidence and three-year outcome in Liverpool. *British Journal of Psychiatry* 161, 230–9.

Da Prada M, Kettler R, Keller HH et al. (1989) Neurochemical profile of moclobemide, a short-acting and reversible inhibitor of monoamine oxidase type A. *Journal of Pharmacology and Experimental Therapeutics* 248, 400–13.

De Vanna M, Kummer J, Agnoli A et al. (1990) Moclobemide compared with second-generation antidepressants in elderly people. *Acta Psychiatrica Scandinavica* Suppl. 360, 64–6.

Dollery C (ed.) 1991 *Therapeutic Drugs* p. L53. Edinburgh, Churchill Livingstone.

Doogan DP and Caillard V (1988) Sertraline: a new antidepressant. *Journal of Clinical Psychiatry* 49, 46–51.

Dorman T (1992) Sleep and paroxetine: a comparison with manserin in elderly depressed patients. *International Clinical Psychopharmacology* 6(Suppl. 4), 53–58.

Dunner DL, Cohn JB, Walshe T et al. (1992) Two combined, multicenter double-blind studies of paroxetine and doxepin in geriatric patients with major depression. *Journal of Clinical Psychiatry* 52 (2, suppl.) 57–60.

Emery G (1981) Cognitive therapy with the elderly. In Hollon SD and Bedrosian RC (eds) *New Directions in Cognitive Therapy*. New York, Guilford.

Fairbairn AF, George K and Dorman T (1989) Lofepramine versus dothiepin in the treatment of depression in elderly patients. *British Journal of Clinical Practice* 43, 55–60.

Falk WE, Rosenbaum JE, Otto MW et al. (1989) Fluoxetine versus trazodone in depressed geriatric patients. *Journal of Geriatric Psychiatry and Neurology* 2, 208–14.

Feighner JP (1983) The new generation of antidepressants. *Journal of Clinical Psychiatry* 44, 49–55.

Feighner JP and Cohn JB (1985) Double-blind comparative trials of fluoxetine and doxepin in geriatric patients with major depressive disorder. *Journal of Clinical Psychiatry* 46, 20–5.

Figiel GS, Krishnan KRR and Doraiswamy PM (1990) Subcortical structural changes in ECT-induced delirium. *Journal of Geriatric Psychiatry and Neurology* 3, 172–6.

Finch EJL and Katona CLE (1989) Lithium augmentation of refractory depression in old age. *International Journal of Geriatric Psychiatry* 4, 41–6.

Fraser RM and Glass IB (1978) Recovery from ECT on elderly patients. *British Journal of Psychiatry* 133, 524–8.

Fraser RM and Glass IB (1980) Unilateral and bilateral ECT in elderly patients: a comparative study. *Acta Psychiatrica Scandinavica* 62, 13–31.

Freeman CRL (1993) Electroconvulsive therapy (ECT) and other physical therapies. In Kendell RE and Zealley AK (eds) *Companion to Psychiatric Studies* (5th edn). Edinburgh, Churchill Livingstone.

Gallagher DE (1981) Behavioural group therapy with elderly depressives: an experimental study. In: Upper D and Ross S (eds) *Behavioural Group Therapy*. Champaign, Ill., Research Press.

Gallagher DE and Thompson LW (1982) Treatment of major depressive disorder in older adult outpatients with bef psychotherapies. *Psychotherapy Research and Practice* 19, 482–90.

Gallagher DE and Thompson LW (1983) Effectiveness of psychotherapy for both endogenous and nonendgenous depression in older adults. *Journal of Gerontology* 38, 307–12.

Gaspar D and Samarasinghe LA (1982) ECT in psychogeriatric practice—a study of risk factors, indications and outcome. *Comprehensive Psychiatry* 23, 170–5.

Georgotas A, Friedman E, McCarthy M et al. (1983) Resistant geriatric depressions and therapeutic response to monoamine oxidase inhibitors. *Biological Psychiatry* 18, 195–205.

Georgotas A, McCue RE, Cooper TB et al. (1989) Factors affecting the delay of anti-depressant effect in responders to nortriptyline and phenelzine. *Psychiatry Research* **28**, 1–9.

Georgotas A, McCue RE Friedman E et al. (1987) The response of depressive symptoms to nortriptyline, phenelzine and placebo. *British Journal of Psychiatry* **151**, 102–6.

Georgotas A, McCue RE, Hapworth W et al. (1986) Comparative efficacy and safety of MAOIs versus TCAs in treating depression in the elderly. *Biological Psychiatry* **21**, 1155–66.

Gerner R, Estabrook W, Steuer J et al. (1980) Teatment of geriatric depression with trazodone, imipramine and placebo: a double-blind study. *Journal of Clinical Psychiatry* **41**, 216–20.

Gerson SC, Plotkin DA and Jarvik LF (1988) Antidepressant drug studies 1946 to 1986: empirical evidence for aging patients. *Journal of Clinical Psychopharmacology* **8**, 311–22.

Ghose K and Sedman E (1987) A double-blind comparison of the pharmacodynamic effects of single doses of lofepramine, amitriptyline and placebo in elderly subjects. *European Journal of Clinical Pharmacology* **33**, 505–9.

Ghose K and Spragg BP (1989) Pharmacokinetics of lofepramine and amitriptyline in elderly healthy subjects. *International Clinical Psychopharmacology* **4**, 201–15.

Gold L and Chiarella CJ (1944) The prognostic value of clinical findings in cases treated with electric shock. *Journal of Nervous and Mental Disease* **100**, 577–83.

Hamilton M (1960) A rating scale for depression. *Journal of Neurology, Neurosurgery and Psychiatry* **23**, 56–62.

Hartman C and Lazarus LW (1992) Psychotherapy with elderly depressed patients. *Clinics in Geriatric Medicine* **8**, 355–62.

Hindmarch I and Bhatti JZ (1988) Psychopharmacological effects of sertraline in normal, healthy volunteers. *European Journal of Clinical Pharmacology* **35**, 221–3.

Hindmarch I, Shillingford J and Shillingford C (1990) The effects of sertraline on psycho-motor performance in elderly volunteers. *Journal of Clinical Psychiatry* **51**, 34–6.

Hobson RF (1953) Prognostic factors in electric convulsive therapy. *Journal of Neurology, Neurosurgery and Psychiatry* **16**, 275–81.

Hutchinson DR, Tong S, Moon CAL et al. (1991) A double blind study in general practice to compare the efficacy and tolerability of paroxetine and amitriptyline in depressed elderly patients. *British Journal of Clinical Research* **2**, 43–7.

Jesse H-J, Jessel I and Wegener G (1981) Therapy for depressive elderly patients: lofepramine and amitriptyline tested under doule-blind conditions. *Zeitschrift für Allgemeinmedizin* **57**, 784–7.

Johnstone ET, Deakin JF, Lawler P et al. (1980) The Northwick Park electroconvulsive therapy trial. *Lancet* **ii**, 1317–20.

Kanba S, Matsumoto K, Nibuya M et al. (1992) Nortriptyline response in elderly depressed patients. *Progress in Neuropsychopharmacology and Biological Psychiatry* **16**, 301–9.

Karlinsky H and Shulman K (1984) The clinical use of electroconvulsive therapy in old age. *Journal of the American Geriatrics Society* **32**, 183–6.

Katona CLE (1991) Refractory epression. In Freeman HL (ed.) *The Uses of Fluoxetine In Clinical Practice.* London, Royal Society of Medicine.

Katona CLE, Aldridge CR, Roth M and Hyde J (1987) The D.S.T. and outcome prediction in patients receiving E.C.T. *British Journal of Psychiatry* **150**, 315–19.

Katona CLE and Finch EJL (1990) Lithium augmentation for refractory depression in old age. In Amsterdam J (ed.) *Refractory Depression.* New York, Raven Press.

Katz IR, Simpson GM, Curlik SM et al. (1990) Pharmacologic treatment of major depression for elderly patients in residential care settings. *Journal of Clinical Psychiatry* **51** (7, suppl.), 41–7.

Kaye CM, Haddock RE, Langley PF et al. (1989) A review of the metabolism and pharmacokinetics of paroxetine in man. *Acta Psychiatrica Scandinavica* **80**, 60–75.

Kelleher K (1992) The afternoon of life: Jung's view of the tasks of the second half of life. *Perspectives in Psychiatric Care* **28**, 25–8.

Kelly GA (1955) *The Psychology of Personal Constructs* (2 vols). New York, Norton.

Kivela S-L, Pahkala K and Laippala P (1988) Prevalence of depression in an elderly population in Finland. *Acta Psychiatrica Scandinavica* **78**, 401–13.

Kushnir SL (1986) Lithium-antidepressant combinations in the treatment of depressed, physically ill geriatric patients. *American Journal of Psychiatry* **143**, 378–9.

Lafferman J, Solomon K and Ruskin P (1988) Lithium augmentation for treatment-resistant depression in the elderly. *Journal of Geriatric Psychiatry and Neurology* **1**, 49–52.

Lam DH and Power MJ (1991) A questionnaire designed to assess roles and goals: a preliminary study. *British Journal of Medical Psychology* **64**, 359–73.

Letemendia FJJ, Delva NJ, Rodenburg M et al. (1993) Therapeutic advantage of bifrontal electrode placement in ECT. *Psychological Medicine* **23**, 349–60.

Levin Y, Elizur A and Korczyn AD (1987) Physostigmine improves ECT-induced memory disturbances. *Neurology* **37**, 871–5.

Lipsey JR, Robinson RG, Pearlson GD et al. (1984) Nortriptyline treatment of post-stroke depression: a double-blind study. *Lancet* **i**, 297–300.

Lovestone S (1993) Cognitive therapy with the elderly depressed: a rational and efficacious approach? In Levy R, Howard R and Burns A (eds) *Treatment and Care in Old Age Psychiatry*. Petersfield, Wrightson Biomedical Publishing.

Lucas RA and Osborne DJ (1986) The disposition of fluoxetine and norfluoxetine in elderly patients with depressive illness compared to younger subjects. In *Proceedings of 16th CINP Congress, Puerto Rico*.

Macdonald AJD (1986) Do general practitioners 'miss' depression in elderly patients? *British Medical Journal* **292**, 1365–7.

McNeil JK, LeBlanc EM and Joyner M (1991) The effect of exercise on depressive symptoms in the moderately depressed elderly. *Psychology and Aging* **6**, 487–8.

Magni G, Fisman M and Helmes E (1988) Clinical correlates of ECT resistant depression in the elderly. *Journal of Clinical Psychiatry* **49**, 405–7.

Maguire K, Pereira A and Tiller J (1991) Moclobemide pharmacokinetics in depressed patients: lack of age effect. *Human Psychopharmacology* **6**, 249–52.

Marmar CR, Gaston L, Gallagher D and Thompson LW (1989) Alliance and outcome in late-life depression. *Journal of Nervous and Mental Disease* **177**, 464–72.

Maynard A (1993) Cost management: the economist's viewpoint. *British Journal of Psychiatry* **163** (suppl. 20), 7–13.

Meredith CH, Feighner JP and Hendrickson G (1984) A double-blind comparative evaluation of the efficacy and safety of nomifensine, imipramine and placebo in depressed geriatric outpatients. *Journal of Clinical Psychiatry* **45**, 73–7.

Miller MD, Pollock BG, Rifai AH et al. (1991) Longitudinal analysis of nortriptyline side effects in elderly depressed patients. *Journal of Geriatric Psychiatry and Neurology* **4**, 226–30.

Mintz J, Steuer J and Jarvik L (1981) Psychotherapy with depressed elderly patients: research considerations. *Journal of Consulting and Clinical Psychology* **49**, 542–8.

Montgomery SA and Asberg M (1979) A new depression scale designed to be sensitive to change. *British Journal of Psychiatry* **134**, 382–9.

Morris RG and Morris LW (1991) Cognitive and behavioural approaches with the depressed elderly. *International Journal of Geriatric Psychiatry* **6**, 407–13.

Moskowitz H and Burns MM (1986) Cognitive performance in geriatric subjects after acute treatment with antidepressants. *Neuropsychobiology* **15**, 38.

Mullan E, D'Ath P, Katona PM and Katona CLE (1994) Detection, fitness for treatment, and management of depression in elderly primary care attenders. Submitted for publication.

Mulsant BH, Rosen J, Thornton JE and Zubenko GS (1991) A prospective naturalistic study of electroconvulsive therapy in late-life depression. *Journal of Geriatric Psychiatry and Neurology* 4, 3–13.

Old Age Depression Interest Group (1993) How long should the elderly take anti-depressants? A double-blind placebo-controlled study of continuation/prophylaxis therapy with dothiepin. *British Journal of Psychiatry* 162, 175–82.

Phanjoo AL, Wonnacott S and Hodgson A (1991) Double-blind comparative multicentre study of fluvoxamine and mianserin in the treatment of major depressive episode in elderly people. *Acta Psychiatrica Scandinavica* 83, 476–9.

Rahman MK, Akhtar MJ, Savla NC et al. (1991) A double-blind, randomised comparison of fluvoxamine with dothiepin in the treatment of depression in elderly patients. *British Journal of Clinical Practice* 45, 255–258.

Raskind M (1984) Electroconvulsive therapy in the elderly. *Journal of the American Geriatrics Society* 32, 177–8.

Rockwell E, Lam RW and Zisook S (1988) Antidepressant drug studies in the elderly. *Psychiatric Clinics of North America* 11, 215–33.

Sackeim HA, Decina P, Prohovnik I et al. (1986) Dosage, seizure threshold and the antidepressant efficacy of electroconvulsive therapy. *Annals of the New York Academy of Sciences* 462, 398–410.

Sackeim H, Decina P, Prohovnik I and Malitz S (1987) Seizure threshold in electro-convulsive therapy. *Archives of General Psychiatry* 44, 355–60.

Shapiro AK, Dussik KT, Tolentino JC et al. (1960) A 'browsing' double blind study of iproniazid in geriatric patients. *Diseases of the Nervous System* 21, 286–7.

Sjogren C (1980) The pharmacological profile of lofpramine: a new antidepressant drug. *Neuropharmacoloqy* 19, 1213–14.

Sommer BR, Satlin A, Friedman L and Cole JO (1989) Glycopyrrolate versus atropine in post-ECT amnesia in the elderly. *Journal of Geriatric Psychiatry and Neurology* 2, 18–21.

Steuer JL, Mintz J, Hammen CL et al. (1984) Cognitive behavioural and psychodynamic group psychotherapy in treatment of geriatric depession. *Journal of Consulting and Clinical Psychology* 52, 180–9.

Stoudemire A, Hill CD, Morris R et al. (1991) Cognitive outcome following tricyclic and electroconvulsive treatment of major depression in the elderly. *American Journal of Psychiatry* 148, 1336–40.

Thompson LW, Gallagher D and Breckenridge JS (1987) Comparative effectiveness of the psychotherapies for depressed elders. *Journal of Consulting and Clinical Psychology* 53, 385–90.

Tiller J, Maguire K and Davies B (1990) A sequential double-blind controlled study of moclobemide and mianserin in elderly depressed patients. *International Journal of Geriatric Psychiatry* 5, 199–204.

Treliving LR (1989) The use of psychodynamics in understanding elderly in-patients. *Psychoanalytic Psychotherapy* 3, 225–33.

Viney LL, Benjamin YN and Preston CA (1990) An evaluation of personal construct therapy for the elderly. *British Journal of Medical Psychology* 62, 35–41.

Wakelin JS (1986) Fluvoxamine in the treatment of the older depressed patient: double-blind placebo-controlled data. *International Clinical Psychopharmacology* 1, 221–30.

Weiner RD (1982) The role of electroconvulsive therapy in the treatment of depression in the elderly. *Journal of the American Geriatrics Society* 30 710–12.

Weiner RD, Rodgers HJ, Davidson JRT et al. (1986) Effects of stimulus parameters on cognitive side effects. *Annals of the New York Academy of Sciences* **462**, 315–25.
Wilkinson DG (1993) ECT in the elderly. In Levy R, Howard R and Burns A (eds) *Treatment and Care in Old Age Psychiatry*. Petersfield, Wrightson Biomedical Pubishling.
Woodhouse K (1992) The pharmacology of major tranquillisers in the elderly. In Katona C and Levy R (eds) *Delusions and Hallucinations in Old Age*. London, Gaskell.
Yesavage JA, Brink TL, Rose TL and Lum O (1983) Development and validation of a geriatric depression screening scale: a preliminary report. *Journal of Psychiatric Research* **17**, 37–49.
Zerhusen JD, Boyle K and Wilson W (1991) Out of the darkness: group cognitive therapy for the elderly. *Journal of Psychosocial Nursing* **29**, 16–20.
Zung WWK (1965) A self-rating depression scale. *Archives of General Psychiatry* **12**, 63–70.

8 The Prognosis of Depression in Old Age

OVERALL OUTCOME

In a seminal early paper, Roth (1955) followed up elderly subjects six months and two years after their inpatient admission to Graylingwell Hospital. By using a precise diagnostic classification, he was able to demonstrate clear differences in prognosis between subjects with affective psychoses (mainly depression), late paraphrenia, acute confusional states and 'senile' and 'arteriosclerotic' dementia. In particular, he was able to show that subjects with affective disorders in old age, though not having the invariably poor outcome of the dementias, nonetheless have a considerable risk of chronicity and, in those initially recovering, a high relapse rate. The replications of Roth's retrospective inpatient studies by Blessed and Wilson (1982) and by Christie (1982) confirmed that, in patients treated in the late 1970s, affective disorder continued to carry a relatively poor prognosis. This was reflected both in the two-year mortality of up to 24% (Christie 1982) and the fact that, in the Blessed and Wilson (1982) study, 21% of subjects were inpatients at the time of two-year follow-up. Similar findings for the late 1980s, again using the same methodology, have been reported by Christie and Wood (1990). In a somewhat longer follow-up, averaging three years, of depressed patients originally admitted under his care, Post (1972), reported that only one in five had made a lasting recovery; nearly two-thirds had had at least one relapse or persisting symptoms; and 12% had failed to recover at all.

Relatively poor prognosis is also reported in studies of subjects initially presenting with depression earlier in life but followed up into old age. Angst (1981) reported on 406 patients with affective disorders who were admitted to the Burgholzli Hospital in Zurich between 1959 and 1963 and who were studied prospectively at five-year intervals until 1980. Thirty-seven per cent of unipolar depressives and 15% of those with bipolar illnesses were relapse free during the 20-year follow-up period. Unipolar subjects with early onset of illness and bipolar subjects had a relapse rate of about 25% after the age of 65, whereas late onset unipolars had a relapse rate of over 40% until age 74 which then fell to 25%. Angst emphasised that none of his subjects received lithium prophylaxis, but the use of other drugs or ECT was not specified and no information was given on other prognostic features or on mortality rate.

Ciompi (1969) studied a cohort of patients admitted to the Lausanne University Psychiatric Hospital aged less than 65 and followed up to 1963 when they were aged between 66 and 90, with length of follow-up ranging between 1 and 52 years. A total of 555 subjects had been admitted with depressive illnesses and 97% were retraced. The average duration of follow-up of these subjects was 20.5 years. It was concluded that depressive symptomatology became gradually less severe in the majority of patients, one-third of whom had no relapse after the age of 65 and another third had less frequent and less severe episodes in old age than previously. One-third, however, exhibited chronic depressive symptoms in old age and there was a tendency for somatised depressive symptoms to replace self-accusatory depressive ideas. Even in those subjects with relatively good outcomes, the occurrence of chronic minor affective symptoms was commonplace. 'More than half of our former depressed patients showed, in senescence, symptoms such as general dissatisfaction, despair, mistrust, demanding behaviour, hypochondria and anxiety. This was associated with decreases in vitality, interests, activities and social contacts. Only 11% were really well adjusted and completely free from all kinds of mental disorders.'

The lack of any clear improvement in prognosis since the late 1940s, when Roth's original cohort was studied, is a cause of both surprise and concern, since one would have expected the routine availability of antidepressant drugs and the development of more comprehensive community supports for the elderly mentally ill to have had some beneficial impact. Equally pessimistic reports from community referrals to psychiatric services have been reported by Murphy (1983). In this study, one-year follow-up revealed that only just over one-third had made a lasting recovery and half had either relapsed or had continuous symptoms. One possible explanation, suggested by Post (1972), is that changes in psychiatric practice in the 1960s, particularly the availability of antidepressants, had led to a higher proportion of elderly depressed patients being treated by primary care physicians without hospital referral. Sixty-one per cent of Post's (1972) cohort had received treatment for their current depression before admission, compared with only 15% in a previous cohort collected by the same author in around 1950 (Post 1962).

Cole (1990) systematically reviewed studies published between 1980 and 1989 in which samples of at least 25 patients with a minimum age of 60 were followed up for at least one year. He was able to identify 10 studies, involving a total of 990 subjects. The combined results showed that although about 25% of subjects developed chronic depression, at least 60% remained well or had relapses with recovery. The more recent of these studies in which clear outcome categories are identified (as well as those published since his review) are summarised in Table 8.1, showing very similar overall outcome figures. The results of these studies are discussed in more detail below.

Baldwin and Jolley (1986), attempted to replicate the findings of Murphy (1983) at one year and of Post (1972) at three years in a retrospective sample. Their one-year recovery rate was nearly 60%, but by three years the overall prognosis

Table 8.1 Recent prognostic studies of depression in old age

	n	Age cut-off (mean)	Diagnostic criteria	Length of follow-up	Well	Relapsed	Continuous illness	Dead
Baldwin and Jolley (1986)	100	≥65 (74)	Feighner	1 year	58	15	18	8
Burvill et al. (1991)	103	>60 (71)	DSM III	1 year	47	18	24	11
Magni et al. (1988b)	64‡	>60 (68)	DSM III	6–24 months	31	\{ 69 \}		0
Kivela et al. (1991)	42*	>60 (73)	DSM III	15 months	45	12	14	14
	199†	>60 (71)		15 months	40	4	42	10
Meats et al. (1991)	56	≥65 (75)	Feighner	1 year	68	12	4	16
Hinrichsen (1992)	127	≥65 (71)	DSM III	1 year	49	23	28	—
Copeland et al. (1992)	107	≥65 (—)	AGECAT	3 years	41	\{ 32 \}		23

* Major depression.
† Dysthymia.
‡ All affective disorders and adjustment disorder with depressed mood.

was almost identical to that in Post's (1972) study. Jolley's group (Meats et al. 1991) have recently replicated their findings in a study in which one-year outcome was compared between consecutively admitted depressed subjects divided into elderly (age >65; n = 56) and younger (n = 24) groups. Outcome in the elderly group was almost identical to that reported by Baldwin and Jolley (1986), and significantly better than in the younger subjects (68% vs 50% 'well' and 16% vs 41% with 'poor' outcome at one year).

Very similar findings have been reported by Hinrichsen (1992), who compared one-year outcome in a consecutive series of elderly depressed inpatients with those of a previously published cohort of patients of mixed age (Keller and Shapiro 1981). Outcome in the elderly group (63% much or very much improved at one year; 72% recovered from the original episode, of whom 23% suffered at least one relapse) was similar both to that in their comparison group of younger subjects and to that in the studies by Jolley's group. Burvill et al. (1991) followed up 103 elderly depressed patients, mostly inpatients. Their results are intermediate between those of Murphy (1983) and Baldwin and Jolley (1986). Forty-seven per cent of subjects had a good outcome in terms of being well at follow-up (whether or not initial recovery had been followed by one or more relapses). Using the more restrictive criterion of lasting recovery, 32% did well.

Two studies have obtained detailed clinical information at follow-up from subjects initially identified by epidemiological survey. Kivela et al. (1991) reported on 42 subjects with DSM III (American Psychiatric Association 1980) major depression and 199 with dysthymia, followed up for 15 months. Good outcome was reported in 45% of those with major depression and 40% of the dysthymics. Mortality was 14% and 10%, respectively, and 14% of the major depression group (but only 3% of the dysthymics) had developed dementia. Copeland et al. (1992) carried out a three-year follow-up study of a sample of 123 subjects with depression (and a further 114 sub-cases), identified from a community sample of 1070 elderly people living in the community. Follow-up information was available on 77 cases and 72 sub-cases, and revealed that 23% of the cases (compared with 21% of non-cases) had died and, of the remainder, 31% were depressed when seen again and a further 13% had improved but were still sub-cases of depression. Among the sub-cases, 17% had died, 18% had become cases and 13% were again sub-cases of depression; 5% of depression cases and 2% of sub-cases had developed dementia.

Cole (1990) evaluated the validity of the studies he reviewed in terms of the nature of the cohort studied, the description of referral pattern, the adequacy of follow-up, the criteria for and assessment of outcome and the degree of adjustment for extraneous prognostic factors. He found that, without exception, the studies suffered from one or more major methodological flaws. Similar conclusions can be reached for the more recent studies summarised in Table 8.1. All the studies (with the exception of Kivela et al. 1991 and Copeland et al. 1992) failed to examine epidemiologically representative samples. Criteria both for diagnosis and outcome were variable, objective outcome criteria were hardly ever used, and outcome assessment (again with the exception of Copeland et al. 1992) was not stated to be blind. The studies also varied very widely in the extent to which extraneous prognostic factors were examined or allowed for.

Methodological problems were particularly evident in the most pessimistic of the studies in Cole's review. Magni et al. (1988b), in a study of 94 elderly depressed referrals to an outpatient service, found that at follow-up a mean of 15 months after referral, less than one-third recovered and remained in good health and the remainder had more or less disabling chronic symptoms. However, the follow-up rate was low (64/94) and subjects studied ranged widely in diagnosis, ranging from adjustment disorder with depressed mood through dysthymic disorder to atypical bipolar disorder. Only 14 subjects had major depression.

Despite these very major limitations, the consistency of overall findings is striking. Cole's review also confirms the suggestion that, although the short-term prognosis may be relatively good, longer follow-up none the less reveals high relapse rates. In Cole's combined data, those studies lasting two years or less showed that 43.7% of subjects were well at follow-up, but in studies lasting longer than two years, that figure fell to 27.4%, the relapse rate going up from 15.8% to 34.2%. Cole noted, however, that in both the short-term and long-term follow-up groups, about 60% of subjects either remained well or had relapses with recovery.

In view of the methodological problems he identified, Cole (1990) made a number of recommendations that form a helpful guide to those contemplating new prognostic studies. Subjects should be identified from community rather than hospital or clinic populations; explicit diagnostic and severity criteria should be defined; possible prognostic factors should be described at the outset using validated criteria; outcome should be assessed using specific and independent measures; and reliability should be established for all measures used.

MORTALITY

A further feature that emerges from several of these studies is a high mortality rate. It appears from the studies summarised in Table 8.1 that the overall mortality at one year is about 12%. This is higher than would be expected, though rigorous comparison with age- and sex-adjusted population norms is difficult because of the variable length of follow-up.

In a detailed report with a longer follow-up period (four years) and focusing on the comparison in mortality rates in elderly depressed subjects compared with matched controls, Murphy et al. (1988) reported an overall mortality in the depressed patients of 34%. This was higher in men (42%) than in women (31%), and in both sexes mortality was significantly increased over that in matched controls (control mortality 9% in men and 17% in women). This study also illustrates the problems of drawing firm conclusions from such data. Poor physical health was much commoner in the depressed subjects, both in terms of acute physical illness and chronic health difficulties. Murphy et al. carried out a number of subgroup analyses and found that, although in subjects with the most severe physical illness depression was not associated with higher mortality, depression *was* associated with significantly increased mortality in subjects with either a severe physical health event or major chronic health difficulty, and there was a trend for increased mortality in the depressed subgroups with minor or absent physical health problems. Murphy et al. (1988) concluded that this provided adequate evidence for an independent predictive effect of depression on mortality.

There does not appear to be any consistent explanation for the excess mortality in depressed elderly subjects. In the study by Ciompi (1969), the reduction in life expectancy in a sample of depressed subjects followed up into old age (5.1% reduction in men and 7.6% in women) was accounted for almost completely by a 7–8 times higher suicide rate in depressed subjects than in the general population. In contrast, a large (n = 898) study of depression and mortality in residents of nursing homes and sheltered accommodation (Parmelee et al. 1992) found that, while mortality at 18 months was higher in subjects with baseline depression, the excess was attributable entirely to the association between depression and physical ill health.

Other community studies fail to confirm an excess mortality associated with depression in old age. Fredman et al. (1989) used the DIS interview and a computer algorithm to determine DSM III (American Psychiatric Association 1980) diagnoses (with a one-year rather than two-year duration criterion for dysthymia) and symptom count measures of severity in 1606 subjects. No significant relationship, or even trend, was found between depression and mortality. Similar negative findings have recently been reported from an even larger community study of 1855 subjects (Thomas et al. 1992). The follow-up period in these studies was, however, relatively short at two years. These results are in keeping with the more psychiatrically detailed community study of Copeland et al. (1992), which found hardly any difference in mortality between depressed and non-depressed subjects, using a longer (three-year) follow-up period.

The relationship between depression and mortality has also been examined in populations defined as physically ill at baseline. Our group has recently found a lack of relationship between depression and mortality in a sample of 119 elderly medical inpatients at one-year follow-up (Finch et al. 1991). In our sample, the mortality in subjects with significant depressive symptoms at initial assessment was 42% and that in the non-depressed 48%. We also did not find any increase in hospital usage by the depressed patients. In contrast, Koenig et al. (1989) reported significantly increased mortality and significantly higher number of days of inpatient care in elderly medical inpatients with major depression compared with non-depressed controls from the same population. As in our study, allowance was made for severity of physical illness as well as diagnosis, but the follow-up period was very short at only five months. The difference in findings is likely to reflect the fact that Koenig et al. (1989) restricted their analysis to patients with relatively severe depressions, only a very small number of whom were identified in our study.

The clearest conclusion to emerge is that the excess mortality associated with depression in old age is seen most clearly in subjects in whom depression is the presenting problem (rather than those identified in community or medical patient epidemiological studies), and tends to emerge 2–4 years after onset, with a relatively favourable very-long-term prognosis. This 'bringing forward' of mortality in the early years after the depressive episode is similar to that reported in bereaved men by Parkes et al. (1969).

Murphy et al. (1988) found that the excess mortality in their depressed subjects was almost entirely by natural causes, mainly cardiovascular and cerebrovascular disease and pneumonia. Only one depressed subject died by suicide but it should be noted that in almost a quarter the cause of death was unknown or unrecorded. The classic very-long-term follow-up study by Ciompi (1969), in contrast, emphasised the importance of suicide as a contributor to the overall high mortality of depression in old age. Ninety-seven per cent of a cohort of 555 depressed patients initially admitted as in patients to psychiatric care in Lausanne were followed up after a mean of over 20 years. Life expectancy was significantly reduced compared with matched controls and this was accounted for almost completely by a suicide rate seven to eight times that in the general population. The more general issues of suicide and parasuicide in old age are discussed in Chapter 4.

It will be apparent from the above that recent studies of prognosis use mortality and persistence of depressive symptoms or diagnosis as their main outcome measures. Cole (1990) has pointed out the imprecision with which outcome criteria such as 'relapse' have been used. More important, these measures alone do scant justice to the comprehensive analysis of prognosis. In particular, relatively little attention has been paid to the relationship between depression and subsequent physical illness, although Murphy (1983) found that new severe health problems occurred in 20% of depressed subjects at one-year follow-up and were significantly commoner in those whose depression had a poor outcome. Blazer et al. (1989) stressed the importance of residual symptomatology in elderly depressed patients and found that in two-thirds of subjects aged 60 and over, early morning anxiety was present one to two years after their hospitalisation with depressive illness. Cognitive impairment at follow-up is reported as rare in elderly depressed patients; 4% of subjects in Murphy's (1983) study developed dementia within one year; this was no more than the expected annual average incidence. Similar findings were reported by Baldwin and Jolley (1986). Surprisingly, quality of life at follow-up in elderly depressed patients has not been formally examined, though the issues involved in such an assessment are well described by Gurland (1992).

CLINICAL PREDICTORS OF PROGNOSIS

SYMPTOM PATTERN

Post (1972) was unable to find any clear association between Newcastle (Carney et al. 1965) Scale-based clinical groupings and outcome, though it should be remembered that, as discussed in Chapter 2, the validity of this scale may be limited in the context of depression in old age. Murphy (1983) used the Present State Examination (PSE; Wing et al. 1974) to distinguish between psychotic and neurotic depression and found no difference in outcome between the two groups. More recently, Magni et al. (1988b), who examined a sample of elderly subjects with a broader range of depressive symptomatology, reported significantly better prognosis in those subjects with DSM III (American Psychiatric Association 1980) adjustment disorder with depressed mood than in those with other diagnoses including major depression. Half the subjects in the adjustment disorder with depressed mood group were, however, lost to follow-up. In contrast, Kivela et al. 1991) found similar one-year outcome in subjects with DSM III major depression and dysthymia, though (not surprisingly, since prior chronicity is part of its definition) chronicity was commoner in the latter group. Georgotas et al. (1989b) examined depressive subtype in a series of patients selected for an antidepressant treatment trial. They found that patients classified as endogenous on the Research Diagnostic Criteria (Spitzer and Endicott 1978) responded faster to the tricyclic antidepressant nortriptyline, but there was no difference between endogenous and non-endogenous subjects in speed of response to the monoamine-oxidase inhibitor phenelzine. It must of course be remembered that DSM III and RDC diagnostic subtypes , like the Newcastle endogenous/non-endogenous distinction and the Feighner criteria (Feighner et al. 1972) used by Baldwin and Jolley (1986) and Meats et al. (1991) were not designed for use in older populations.

Murphy (1983) suggested that the presence of depressive delusions may be more prognostically informative than endogenicity. She found that although there was no difference in one-year outcome between subjects classified as psychotic or neurotic, only one in ten of those with delusional depression had recovered, in contrast to 70% of those without delusions. In contrast, Baldwin (1988), in a comparison between the 24 deluded subjects identified by Baldwin and Jolley (1986) and an individually matched group of non-deluded subjects from the same cohort, reported that delusional depression did not carry a worse prognosis. Burvill et al. (1991) also reported the absence of any significant predictive effect of delusions. Baldwin and Jolley (1986) suggest that these apparently divergent findings may be explicable in terms of the low rate of use of ECT in Murphy's sample. Forty-eight per cent of subjects in Baldwin and Jolley's (1986) sample received ECT, compared with 38% in that of Burvill et al. (1991) and only 16% in that of Murphy (1983). Possible treatment effects on outcome are discussed in detail later in this chapter.

SEVERITY

Murphy (1983) used PSE total symptom scores and intensity and persistence of symptoms to obtain a global rating of severity, and found significantly poorer one-year outcome in subjects with severe illness. This was confirmed by Baldwin and Jolley (1986), who found that almost all of the subjects in their study who became chronically depressed had index Hamilton Depression Rating Scores (Hamilton 1960) of 30 or more. Georgotas et al. (1989b) found that response to antidepressant treatment was slower in patients with more severe illnesses and the same group (Georgotas et al. 1989) found that the relapse rate was also higher in those patients with more severe depression.

COGNITIVE IMPAIRMENT

A number of studies, notably those of Murphy (1983), Murphy et al. (1988) and Baldwin and Jolley (1986), specifically excluded depressed patients with significant cognitive impairment. There has, however, been considerable interest in the prognosis of those patients with 'depressive pseudodementia'. The influential paper by Kral (1983) suggested that most if not all patients with significant but initially reversible cognitive impairment as part of their depressive presentation went on to develop dementia of the Alzheimer type. Kral's findings were recently extended in the report by Kral and Emery (1989), who identified 44 such patients (mean age 76.5 years) with rapid onset of loss of interests, slowing, and poor concentration, memory and orientation, coexistent with severe depression characterised by self-depreciation, guilt, suicidal ideas and loss of appetite. Though all subjects responded well to antidepressant treatment, follow-up for an average of eight years revealed that 89 subsequently developed dementia of the Alzheimer type. Magni et al. (1988b) also found significantly worse prognosis in those depressed patients with 'organic impairment of the central nervous system': only 2 out of 20 patients in the impaired group recovered fully. Less striking but similar findings have been reported by Alexopoulos et al. (1989), who found that 39% of depressed patients with initially reversible dementia developed irreversible dementia within two to four years. In marked contrast, Pearlson et al. (1989) found that at two-year follow-up only 1 of 11 patients with depressive pseudo-dementia went on to develop an unequivocal dementing illness. Baldwin et al. (1993) carried out a systematic comparison of one-year outcome between 32 patients with depressed mood and cerebral pathology and 66 cerebrally intact depressed elderly patients. Outcome in terms of depression was similar in the two groups, though the cognitively impaired sample had a higher mortality (25% vs 12%). In a sample restricted to residents of nursing homes and sheltered accommodation, Parmelee et al. (1991) found depression to be a significant predictor of subsequent cognitive impairment at one-year follow-up, but that cognitive impairment at baseline was not associated with greater likelihood of subsequent depression.

DEMOGRAPHIC FACTORS

Murphy (1983), Baldwin and Jolley (1986) and Herrmann et al. (1989) all found that age did not affect prognosis. A community study by Kennedy et al. (1991), however, found advanced age to be significantly associated with persistence of depression, even after multivariate analysis to allow for the effects of physical ill-health.

There is some evidence that, at least in longer-term follow-up, the prognosis is better in depressed women than in men. Murphy (1983) found no difference in one-year prognosis by sex, but, as discussed earlier in this chapter, mortality at four-year follow-up (Murphy et al. 1988) was much more in excess of that for controls in men than in women. Similarly, Baldwin and Jolley (1986) found that lasting recovery was recorded in only 1 of 21 men compared with 21 of 79 women. This is in contrast with the long-term follow-up data of Lee and Murray (1988) in younger subjects, in which there was no sex difference in relapse rate.

PAST HISTORY AND CT SCAN ABNORMALITY

The possibility that patients with first onset of depression in old age have a particularly poor prognosis has been raised by Jacoby and Levy (1980), who identified a subgroup of patients with onset after the age of 60 who had enlarged ventricles on CT scan and a high mortality. Alexopoulos (1989) has suggested that a subgroup of elderly depressed patients with poor prognosis may have a syndrome characterised by late first onset, ventricular enlargement on CT scan and reversible dementia, all indicating underlying degenerative brain disease.

Systematic studies have, however, provided little evidence in support of the association between late age at first onset and poor prognosis. Georgotas and McCue (1989) found that early relapse (within two months of initial recovery) was commoner in those patients with several previous admissions, but there was no difference in age at first onset between relapsers and non-relapsers. Murphy (1983) reported no difference in one-year outcome between subjects with and without a past history of depression earlier in life, and Baldwin and Jolley (1986) found no association between outcome and past psychiatric history at a follow-up of up to 104 months. A similar lack of relationship between age at first onset and short-term treatment outcome was reported by Greenwald and Kramer-Ginsberg (1988). However, Conwell et al. (1989) found that late onset elderly depressed patients had more residual symptoms at discharge and a significantly greater length of stay in hospital, though not differing in age at index episode. In striking contrast, Magni et al. (1988b) found that good outcome at 6–24-month follow-up was much better in late onset subjects. Unfortunately, Murphy et al. (1988), in the most comprehensive study to date of mortality in elderly depressed patients, did not examine the relationship between age at first onset and four-year mortality.

An historical variable showing a more consistent relationship with outcome than age at first onset is chronicity of the current episode, though this may be difficult to assess because of the frequency with which 'double depression', i.e. an acute depressive episode superimposed on a chronic dysthymia, is seen in old age (Alexopoulos et al. 1989). Murphy (1983) found that although only one-fifth of her subjects had illnesses lasting longer than a year prior to the study, they accounted for more than a quarter of those in the poor outcome group and only 11% of those in the good outcome group. This difference did not, however, reach statistical significance. Baldwin and Jolley (1986) did not find any relationship between duration of illness and outcome, but Georgotas et al. (1988) found that all 11 relapsers among 60 elderly depressed patients in whom maintenance nortriptyline or phenelzine was being evaluated following clinical recovery had had depressions lasting at least two years.

The possible prognostic importance of past history of other psychiatric disorders has received little attention. However, Cook et al. (1991) have reported that in a predominantly elderly sample (minimum age 55) of depressed subject, those with a history of alcohol abuse not only had longer admissions but at follow-up (four years after admission) they had had much more persistent symptoms and more frequent re-admissions. These potentially important findings are made more difficult to interpret by the fact that only 50% of subjects with a past history of alcoholism had remained abstinent during the follow-up period of their depressive illness.

PHYSICAL HEALTH

Several studies have concluded that poor physical health predicts poor outcome of depression in old age. Post (1972) found that disabling physical illness predicted a poor outcome. This was confirmed by Murphy (1983), who found that both chronic health problems (present in 49% of the poor outcome group and in only 29% of those with good outcomes) and acute new physical illness during the follow-up period (29% vs 7%) predicted poor one-year outcome. Murphy et al. (1988) confirmed this in their four-year follow-up, with a 22% mortality in the physically well group but one of nearly 50% in those with severe health events or major chronic health difficulties. They pointed out that, though physical health problems contributed to the excess mortality over controls, depression itself appeared to have an independent influence on mortality. Baldwin and Jolley (1986) also reported results consistent with the above; 91% of patients experiencing a lasting recovery had no active physical pathology on presentation, while 71% of those who remained continuously depressed had had at least one active physical health problem on admission. Similarly, the Old Age Depression Interest Group (1993), in a study with a primary focus on the efficacy of prophylactic antidepressants, found that physical ill health was the most powerful predictor of depressive relapse over a two-year follow-up period. Harris et al. (1988) examined depressive symptomatology on admission and at discharge in a group of 30 elderly patients with severe physical illness and found that persistence of depression was associated with failure of physical rehabilitation. Burvill et al.

(1991), however, found no association between acute or chronic physical illness prior to onset of depression or emergent physical illness during the follow-up period, and Magni et al. (1988b) also found no relationship between physical illness and outcome. It should be noted, however, that the sample studied by Magni et al. was relatively small, and that the same authors (Magni et al. 1988a) when comparing responders and non-responders to ECT found that poor therapeutic response was indeed significantly associated with physical illness during the index episode.

All the above studies have focused on cases identified through psychiatric services. In a more representative sample of subjects identified by community survey, Kennedy et al. (1991) found that worsening health was the most powerful predictor of persisting depression, and improving physical health of its remission.

SOCIAL CIRCUMSTANCES AND LIFE EVENTS

Several studies reviewed by Cole (1990) concluded that marital status and living circumstances were unrelated to outcome. The more recent results of Burvill et al. (1991) are also consistent with this. Murphy (1983) studied the availability of intimate relationships (whose aetiological importance is discussed in Chapter 4) as a potentially more relevant prognostic factor than marital status and living circumstances, but although there was a trend for those with a lack of a confidant to be more frequently in the poor outcome group (54% vat 36%), this was not statistically significant.

A number of studies have focused more specifically on the prognostic effect of recent adverse life events. Murphy (1983) found that severe adverse events in the year prior to onset of the depression did not predict poor prognosis, but that those in the poor outcome group were more likely (24% vs 7%) to have experienced an adverse event in the follow-up year. This finding was more marked when severe personal health events were included (combined rates 14% in the good outcome group and 47% in those with poor outcome). A similar though not statistically significant trend (44% vs 29%) was found for chronic social difficulties. Baldwin and Jolley (1986) also failed to find any relationship between recent adverse life events and prognosis. Burvill et al. (1991), however, found adverse life events in the three months before admission to be predictive of a good outcome. Predictors of persistent depression within the specific context of bereavement have been examined by Gilewski et al. (1991). Poor outcome was associated with significant depressive symptomatology at the time of the bereavement, and with bereavement by suicide.

Krause (1988) found that positive life changes, particularly events associated with expansion of family roles, tended to be associated with an increased sense of well-being and a reduction in depressive symptoms, particularly depressive cognition. This clinical improvement was associated with a reduction in external locus of control orientation. He emphasised that the relationship demonstrated may reflect a causal link opposite in direction to that anticipated in that it may be the improvement in depressive symptomatology that allows for expansion of family roles.

PERSONALITY

Thompson et al. (1988), using the structured interview for DSM III personality disorders (Pfohl et al. 1982), found evidence of apparent abnormality of personality during depressive illness in two-thirds of elderly depressed patients and evidence of personality disorder manifest in the subject's 'typical self' in one-third. They reported that short-term outcome of psychotherapeutic treatment (cognitive therapy, behaviour therapy or brief psychodynamic therapy) was significantly better in those free of any evidence of personality disorder during the episode. There was a non-significant trend towards maintenance of this difference at 12-month follow-up. Very similar findings were reported concerning superiority of response in subjects with no 'typical self' evidence of personality disorder, again with only a non-significant trend towards better outcome apparent at 12 months.

A CAVEAT

It should be borne in mind in interpreting all the above studies examining potential predictors of outcome that, as Burvill et al. (1991) point out, the sample size in all outcome studies to date, including their own, has been inadequate to have the statistical power to detect small but clinically significant relationships with outcome. On this basis they consider it unsurprising that, in their own study, multivariate logistic regression analysis did not enable them to reject the null hypothesis that all the potential predictors examined had a zero relationship with outcome. The difficulty in identifying independent predictors of prognosis is further confounded by the impossibility in naturalistic studies of controlling adequately for treatment factors, and by the complex inter-relationships between factors such as, for example, severity, the presence of delusions and the likelihood of use of ECT.

EFFECTS OF TREATMENT ON PROGNOSIS

Although the many studies reviewed above make it apparent that the prognosis of depression in old age is relatively poor, they also illustrate its variability. The effect of treatment interventions on such variability deserves closer attention than it has yet received. Baldwin and Jolley (1986) have suggested that the better short-term outcome in their subjects than those of Murphy (1983) may be explained by the much higher (48% vs 16%) use of ECT in their cohort. This view is supported by the more recent findings of Godber et al. (1987) who reported a very good overall three-year outcome (59% fully well) in elderly depressed subjects treated with ECT. Similarly, Rubin et al. (1991) in a study of 101 depressed patients aged

64–92 years, 46% of whom received ECT, found that ECT was the single most important variable associated with good immediate outcome.

The undoubted benefits of antidepressant treatment on short-term outcome that have been demonstrated in clinical trials in elderly subjects may not, because of undertreatment, be reflected in the clinical practice seen in community prognostic studies. Copeland et al. (1992) found that their overall poor prognosis was associated with an extremely low detection and treatment rate: only 4% had been treated with antidepressants. Similarly, Iliffe et al. (1991) found that only 6 of the 52 primary care patients they identified by brief clinical interview as depressed had been noted in their GP records to be depressed, and only 3 treated for depression. Also in keeping with this is the report by Macdonald (1986) that though GPs were able, on direct questioning, to identify interview-detected depression in their elderly patients with a high degree of accuracy, they hardly ever either initiated antidepressant treatment or made psychiatric referrals for their depressed elderly subjects.

Even in those elderly patients who failed to respond to initial antidepressant treatment, the judicious use of more invasive pharmacological strategies may improve prognosis. Katona and Finch (1990) demonstrated that lithium augmentation in tricyclic-resistant elderly depressed patients was associated with a good outcome for up to 18 months.

The value of prophylactic antidepressant treatment in preventing relapse has been very inadequately evaluated in elderly subjects. Georgotas et al. (1989a) carried out a placebo-controlled evaluation of maintenance nortriptyline and phenelzine in elderly depressed patients who had responded to antidepressants. Patients on phenelzine had a much lower (13.3%) relapse rate than those on either nortriptyline (53.8%) or placebo (65.2%). The latter two groups did not differ significantly. This study clearly establishes the potential prophylactic usefulness of phenelzine in initial phenelzine responders. The lack of prophylactic efficacy of nortriptyline may in the authors' view, be due to the accumulation of its metabolite 10-hydroxynortriptyline, which increases with age and may interfere with the antidepressant effect of the parent compound. This clearly needs replication. Open studies of continuation fluoxetine and doxepin (Feighner and Cohn 1985) and of sertraline and amitriptyline (Invicta Pharmaceuticals, data on file) suggest that these tricyclic antidepressants and SSRIs appear to be similarly effective in relapse prevention in old age. A recent placebo-controlled study in recovered elderly depressed patients (Old Age Depression Interest Group 1993) has provided more definitive evidence. In 69 patients allocated randomly to receive dothiepin (75 mg/day) or placebo over a two-year period, survival analysis showed relative risk of relapse to be two and a half times greater in the placebo group.

The prophylactic effectiveness of lithium in preventing depressive relapse has been established in a substantial cohort of elderly patients examined retrospectively by Abou-Saleh and Coppen (1983). Though psychosocial interventions have been subjected to still less formal evaluation, they may also be important in reducing risk of depressive relapse in elderly subject. An elegant small study by Ong et al. (1987) found that when elderly depressed inpatients were allocated, following recovery and discharge, to attendance or non-attendance at a psychotherapy support group, six out of ten in the control group required readmission within six months, whereas readmission was not required in any subjects in the active treatment group. Such a finding clearly needs replication in a larger sample.

CONCLUSIONS

Though depression in old age is associated with higher chronicity and mortality than would be found in younger subjects, it seems clear that lasting recovery can be expected in at least 50%. Several factors have been shown with more or less consistency to predict poor outcome. Notable among these are cognitive impairment, physical illness, and the severity and chronicity of the depressive episode itself. The identification of good and poor prognostic groups is of potential value in identifying subjects in whom initial attempts in treatment should be most energetic. This argument is supported by the evidence, admittedly far from adequate as yet, that both acute treatment and systematic prophylaxis (using physical and/or psychosocial methods) can improve prognosis. There is a clear need for further research in which larger samples are studied, clear and agreed outcome criteria are used, and the value of prophylactic interventions systematically evaluated.

REFERENCES

Abou-Saleh MT and Coppen A (1983) The prognosis of depression in old age: the case for lithium therapy. *British Journal of Psychiatry* **143**, 527–8.
Alexopoulos GS (1989) Late-life depression and neurological brain disease. *International Journal of Geriatric Psychiatry* **4**, 187–9.
Alexopoulos GS, Young RC, Abrams RC et al. (1989) Chronicity and relapse in geriatric depression. *Biological Psychiatry* **26**, 551–64.
American Psychiatric Association (1980) *Diagnostic and Statistical Manual of Psychiatric Disorders* (3rd edn). Washington, American Psychiatric Association.
Angst J (1981) Clinical indicators for a prophylactic treatment of depression. *Advances in Biological Psychiatry*, 218–30.
Baldwin RC (1988) Delusional and non-delusional depression in late life: evidence for distinct subtypes. *British Journal of Psychiatry* **152** 39–44.
Baldwin RC, Benbow SM, Marriott A and Tomenson B (1993) Depression in old age. A reconsideration of cerebral disease in relation to outcome. *British Journal of Psychiatry* **163**, 82–90.
Baldwin RC and Jolley DJ (1986) The prognosis of depression in old age. *British Journal of Psychiatry* **149**, 574–83.
Blazer D, Hughes DC and Fowler N (1989) Anxiety as an outcome symptom of depression in elderly and middle-aged adults. *International Journal of Geriatric Psychiatry* **4**, 273–8.

Blessed G and Wilson ID (1982) The contemporary natural history of depression in old age. *British Journal of Psychiatry* 141, 59–67.

Burvill PW, Hall WD, Stampfer HG and Emmerson JP (1991) The prognosis of deprsion in old age. *British Journal of Psychiatry*, 64–71.

Carney MWP, Roth M and Garside RF (1965) The diagnosis of depressive symptoms and the prediction of ECT response. *British Journal of Psychiatry* 114, 659–74.

Christie AB (1982) Changing patterns of mental illness in the elderly. *British Journal of Psychiatry* 140, 154–9.

Christie AB and Wood ERM (1990) Further changes in the pattern of mental illness in the elderly. *British Journal of Psychiatry* 157, 228–31.

Ciompi L (1969) Follow-up studies on the evolution of former neurotic and depressive states in old age: clinical and psychodynamic aspects. *Journal of Geriatric Psychiatry* 3, 90–106.

Cole MG (1990) The prognosis of depression in the elderly. *Canadian Medical Association Journal* 142, 633–9.

Conwell Y, Nelson JC, Kim KM and Mazure CM (1989) Depression in late life: age of onset as marker of a subtype. *Journal of Affective Disorders* 17, 189–95.

Cook BL, Winokur G, Garvey MJ and Beach V (1991) Depression and previous alcoholism in the elderly. *British Journal of Psychiatry* 158, 72–5.

Copeland JR, Davidson IA, Dewey ME et al. (1992) Alzheimer's disease, other dementia, depression and pseudodementia: prevalence, incidence and three-year outcome in Liverpool. *British Journal of Psychiatry* 161, 230–9.

Feighner JP and Cohn JB (1985) Double-blind comparative trials of fluoxetine and doxepin in geriatric patients with major depressive disorder. *Journal of Clinical Psychiatry* 46, 20–5.

Feighner JP, Robins E, Guze SB et al. (1972) Diagnostic criteria for us in psychiatric research. *Archives of General Psychiatry* 26, 57–63.

Finch EJL, Ramsay RL, Wright P et al. (1991) Maladies psychiatriques et leurs suites parmi des vieillards hospitalisés d'urgence pour soins medicaux: étude de contrôle a long terme. *Psychologie Medicale* 23, 735–40.

Fredman L, Schoenback VJ, Kaplan BH et al. (1989) The association between depressive symptoms and mortality among older participants in the Epidemiologic Catchment Area–Piedmont health survey. *Journal of Gerontology: Social Sciences* 44, S149–56.

Georgotas A and McCue RE (1989) Relapse of depressed patients after effective continuation therapy. *Journal of Affective Disorders* 17, 159–64.

Georgotas A, McCue RE, Cooper TB et al. (1988) How effective and safe is continuation therapy in elderly depressed patients? Factors affecting relapse rate. *Archives of General Psychiatry* 45, 929–32.

Georgotas A, McCue RE and Cooper TB (1989a) A placebo-controlled comparison of nortriptyline and phenelzine in maintenance therapy of elderly depressed patients. *Archives of General Psychiatry* 46, 783–5.

Georgotas A, McCue RE, Cooper TB et al. (1989b) Factors affecting the delay of anti-depressant effect in responders to nortriptyline and phenelzine. *Psychiatry Research* 28, 1–9.

Gilewski MJ, Farberow NL, Gallagher DE and Thompson LW (1991) Interaction of depression and bereavement on mental health in the elderly. *Psychology and Aging* 6, 67–75.

Godber C, Rosenvinge H, Wilkinson D et al. (1987) Depression in old age: prognosis after ECT. *International Journal of Geriatric Psychiatry* 2, 19–24.

Greenwald BS and Kramer-Ginsberg E (1988) Age at onset in geriatric depression: relationship to clinical variables. *Journal of Affective Disorders* 15, 61–8.

Gurland B (1992) The impact of depression on quality of life of the elderly. *Clinics in Geriatric Medicine*, 377–86.

Hamilton M (1960) A rating scale for depression. *Journal of Neurology, Neurosurgery and Psychiatry* 23, 56–62.

Harris RE, Mion LC, Patterson MB and Frengley JD (1988) Severe illness in older patients: the association between depressive disorders and functional dependency during the recovery phase. *Journal of the American Geriatric Society* 36, 890–6.

Herrmann N, Lieff S and Silberfield M (1989) The effect of age of onset on depression in the elderly. *Journal of Geriatric Psychiatry and Neurology* 2, 182–7.

Hinrichsen GA (1992) Recovery and relapse from major depressive disohder in the elderly. *American Journal of Psychiatry* 149, 1575–9.

Iliffe S, Haines A, Gallivan S et al. (1991) Assessment of elderly people in general practice 1. Social circumstancs and mental state. *British Journal of General Practice* 41, 9–12.

Jacoby RJ and Levy R (1980) Computed tomography in the elderly: 3. Affective disorder. *British Journal of Psychiatry* 136, 270–5.

Katona CLE and Finch EJL (1990) Lithium augmentation for refractory depression in the elderly. In Amsterdam J (ed.). *Refractory Depression*. New York, Raven Press.

Keller MB and Shapiro RW (1981) Major depressive disorder: initial results from a one-year naturalistic follow-up study. *Journal of Nervous and Mental Disease* 169, 761–7.

Kennedy GJ, Kelman HR and Thomas C (1991) Persistence and remission of depressive symptoms in late life. *American Journal of Psychiatry* 148, 174–8.

Kivela S-L, Pahkala K and Eronen A (1991) A one-year prognosis of dysthymic disorder and major depression in old age. *International Journal of Geriatric Psychiatry* 6, 81–7.

Koenig HG, Shelp F, Goli V et al. (1989) Survival and health care utilization in elderly medical inpatients with major depression. *Journal of the American Geriatrics Society* 37, 599–606.

Kral VA (1983) The relationship between senile dementia (Alzheimer type) and depression. *Canadian Journal of Psychiatry* 28, 304–6.

Kral VA and Emery OB (1989) Long-term follow-up of depressive pseudodementia of the aged. *Canadian Journal of Psychiatry* 34, 445–6.

Krause N (1988) Positive life events and depressive symptoms in older adults. *Behavioral Medicine* 14, 101–12.

Lee AS and Murray RM (1988) The long-term outcome of Maudsley depressives. *British Journal of Psychiatry* 153, 741–51.

Macdonald AJD (1986) Do general practitioners 'miss' depression in elderly patients? *British Medical Journal* 292, 1365–7.

Magni G, Fisman M and Helmes E (1988a) Clinical correlates of ECT-resistant depression in the elderly. *Journal of Clinical Psychiatry* 49, 405–7.

Magni G, Palazzolo O and Bianchin G (1988b) The course of depression in elderly outpatients. *Canadian Journal of Psychiatry* 33, 21–4.

Meats P, Timol M and Jolley D (1991) Prognosis of depression in the elderly. *British Journal of Psychiatry* 159, 659–63.

Murphy E (1983) The prognosis of depression in old age. *British Journal of Psychiatry* 142, 111–19.

Murphy E, Smith R, Lindesay J and Slattery J (1988) Increased mortality rates in late-life depression. *British Journal of Psychiatry* 152, 347–53.

Old Age Depression Interest Group (1993) How long should the elderly take anti-depressants? A double-blind placebo-controlled study of continuation/prophylaxis therapy with dothiepin. *British Journal of Psychiatry* 162, 175–82.

Ong YK, Martineau F, Lloyd C and Robbins I (1987) A support group for the depressed elderly. *International Journal of Geriatric Psychiatry* **2**, 119–23.

Parkes CM, Benjamin B and Fitzgerald RG (1969) Broken heart: a statistical study of increased mortality among widowers. *British Medical Journal* **1**, 740.

Parmelee PA, Katz IR and Lawton MP (1992) Depression and mortality among institutionalised aged. *Journal of Gerontology* **47**, P3–10.

Parmelee PA, Kleban MH, Lawton MP and Katz IR (1991) Depression and cognitive change among institutionalised aged. *Psychology and Aging* **6**, 504–11.

Pearlson GD, Rabins PV, Kim WS et al. (1989) Structural brain CT changes and cognitive deficits in elderly depressives with and without reversible dementia ('pseudodementia'). *Psychological Medicine* **19**, 573–84.

Pfohl B, Stangl D and Zimmerman M (1982) *Structured Clinical Interview for DSM-III Personality Disorders.* Iowa, University of Iowa.

Post F (1962) *The Significance of Affective Symptoms in Old Age.* Maudsley Monographs 10. London, Oxford University Press.

Post F (1972) The management and nature of depressive illnesses in late life: a follow-through study. *British Journal Psychiatry* **121**, 393–404.

Roth M (1955) The natural history of mental disorder in old age. *Journal of Mental Science* **101**, 281–301.

Rubin EH, Kinscherf DA and Wehrman SA (1991) Response to treatment of depression in the old and very old. *Journal of Geriatric Psychiatry and Neurology* **4**, 65–70.

Spitzer RL and Endicott J (1978) *Research Diagnostic Criteria for a Selected Group of Functional Disorders* (3rd edn). New York, New York State Psychiatric Institute.

Thomas C, Kelman HR, Kennedy GJ et al. (1992) Depressive symptoms and mortality in elderly persons. *Journal of Gerontology* **47**, S80–7.

Thompson LW, Gallagher D and Czirr R (1988) Personality disorder and outcome in the treatment of late-life depression. *Journal of Geriatric Psychiatry* **21**, 133–53.

Wing JK, Cooper JE and Sartorius N (1974) *Measurement and Classification of Psychiatric Symptoms.* Cambridge, Cambridge University Press.

9　Future Directions

For all that has been learnt about depression in old age in the past few years there is much we still need to know. A number of research areas appear particularly fruitful. Perhaps still more important, the challenge of providing adequate care for a growing number of older people who become depressed will require considerable changes in public policy as well as medical practice. Areas of particular potential for research and for clinical care will be discussed separately below.

PROMISING AREAS FOR RESEARCH

We still badly need an adequate classification of the depressions of old age. The most promising contenders appear to be the early vs late onset distinction, and an adaptation of the division between severe and mild depressions that takes account of the different pattern of symptoms encountered in old age. Future epidemiological, biological and prognostic studies can all contribute to the validation of a new classificatory system. In the shorter term it will be necessary to discover how the new generation of classificatory systems for mental illness in younger patients (DSM IV, ICD 10) perform in older patients with significant depressive symptomatology.

The availability of portable versions of the Geriatric Mental Status interview makes it much easier for epidemiological studies to share a common system of information gathering and diagnostic decision making. The use of the GMS in a wide variety of settings will make a major contribution to our understanding not only of the epidemiology itself, but of social and cultural contributions to the aetiology of depression in old age.

Biological research should remain a growth industry. In particular, new imaging techniques are likely to be of increasing importance. Magnetic resonance spectroscopy should help bridge the gap between functional and structural imaging. Both single photon emission tomography (SPET) and (despite its great expense) positron emission tomography (PET) are becoming more widely available. They should soon allow the quantification of specific neurotransmitter receptors in the brains of depressed and healthy elderly subjects, and enable the effects of treatments (psychological as well as physical) to be monitored in terms of changes in brain function. Neuro-activation PET and SPET may also help elucidate the changes in brain function underlying the reversible and irreversible changes in cognitive test performance associated with depression in old age. More specific tests of neuroendocrine and monoamine function may also help elucidate the inter-relationships between age and depression-associated abnormalities in these systems.

We still know much less than we should about the efficacy of different treatments for depression in old age. Future studies should recruit large enough samples to examine subjects aged 75 and over (in whom age-related changes in physiological function are particularly important) separately from the 65–74 age group, who resemble the middle-aged much more than they do the very old. Most treatments for depression (both physical and psychological) have not been shown unequivocally to be superior to placebo in an elderly population. The absence of such information renders placebo-controlled trials ethically still permissible and much to be encouraged. The comparative efficacy of psychological and physical treatments also remains almost entirely unknown. Perhaps more fundamentally, treatment trials should attempt to be much more naturalistic in terms of entry criteria and should take into account health-economic and quality-of-life measures as well as changes in depression rating scale scores. This is particularly true in the area of relapse prevention (in which it is also true to say that almost all treatments remain unevaluated).

Management of resistant depression in old age remains far from ideal. Both safer drug strategies for such patients and novel techniques for increasing the 'efficiency' of ECT need to be evaluated in this population.

Finally, despite the large number of recent studies of prognosis, there is still a clear need for future work examining epidemiologically representative samples of sufficient size to allow the influence of inter-related prognostic factors to be teased out.

CLINICAL ISSUES

Despite all our new knowledge about it, depression in old age remains (as I stated at the beginning of this book) common, underdetected and undertreated. The potential benefits of an educational initiative, focused mainly at medical students and the primary care team (which consists of many potentially useful staff apart from the doctors!) would be considerable. Such an initiative would need to undermine ignorance-related therapeutic nihilism. More fundamentally, it should challenge ageist assumptions concerning the inevitability of old age being miserable and the inability of elderly people to change.

At the level of individual case detection, there is good evidence that simple screening tests can add usefully to the ability of primary care and hospital doctors to detect depression in their elderly patients. The use of such instruments should become a matter of routine. It remains, of course, an open question whether the same treatments that work in a minority of severely ill patients fulfilling standard criteria for depression will be as effective in primary care patients identified as depressed by such screening, and indeed whether such patients would be willing to accept treatment. Education about the high prevalence of depression in old age and its potential for treatment needs to be provided for elderly people and their curers as well as to health and social service professionals.

Perhaps the largest nettle to be grasped, however, is the political one. It is clear that poverty, social isolation and poor physical health are among the most important aetiological factors increasing vulnerability to depression in old age. The economic change necessary to provide adequate financial stability and good quality health care to a growing elderly population are enormous. The rising tide of articulate elderly people will have to work closely with those providing medical and social care for their less-fortunate fellow elders to generate the political impetus for such change.

I have every confidence that advances in research will make this book rapidly out of date and I hope that its readers will contribute to that obsolescence. It remains to be seen whether sufficient resources can be generated to enable research progress to be translated into better clinical practice.

Index

Note: Page references in *italics* refer to Figues; those in **bold** refer to Tables

Index compiled by Annette Musker